Color Atlas of
Dermatophytoses
Focus on Superficial Fungal Infections

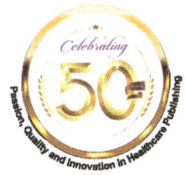

Color Atlas of
Dermatophytoses
Focus on Superficial Fungal Infections

Editor
Jayakar Thomas MD DD MNAMS FRCP FRCPCH PhD DSc

Professor and Head
Department of Dermatology
Sree Balaji Medical College and Hospital
Chennai, Tamil Nadu, India

Co-Editor
Parimalam Kumar MD DD MNAMS FRCP

Professor and Head
Department of Dermatology
Stanley Medical College and Hospital
Chennai, Tamil Nadu, India

Foreword
UR Dhanalakshmi

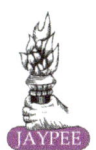

JAYPEE BROTHERS MEDICAL PUBLISHERS
The Health Sciences Publisher
New Delhi | London

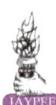 **Jaypee Brothers Medical Publishers (P) Ltd**

Headquarter
Jaypee Brothers Medical Publishers (P) Ltd
4838/24, Ansari Road, Daryaganj
New Delhi 110 002, India
Phone: +91-11-43574357
Fax: +91-11-43574314
Email: jaypee@jaypeebrothers.com

Overseas Office
J.P. Medical Ltd
83 Victoria Street, London
SW1H 0HW (UK)
Phone: +44 20 3170 8910
Fax: +44 (0)20 3008 6180
Email: info@jpmedpub.com

Website: www.jaypeebrothers.com
Website: www.jaypeedigital.com

© 2021, Jaypee Brothers Medical Publishers

The views and opinions expressed in this book are solely those of the original contributor(s)/author(s) and do not necessarily represent those of editor(s) of the book.

All rights reserved. No part of this publication may be reproduced, stored or transmitted in any form or by any means, electronic, mechanical, photocopying, recording or otherwise, without the prior permission in writing of the publishers.

All brand names and product names used in this book are trade names, service marks, trademarks or registered trademarks of their respective owners. The publisher is not associated with any product or vendor mentioned in this book.

Medical knowledge and practice change constantly. This book is designed to provide accurate, authoritative information about the subject matter in question. However, readers are advised to check the most current information available on procedures included and check information from the manufacturer of each product to be administered, to verify the recommended dose, formula, method and duration of administration, adverse effects and contraindications. It is the responsibility of the practitioner to take all appropriate safety precautions. Neither the publisher nor the author(s)/editor(s) assume any liability for any injury and/or damage to persons or property arising from or related to use of material in this book.

This book is sold on the understanding that the publisher is not engaged in providing professional medical services. If such advice or services are required, the services of a competent medical professional should be sought.

Every effort has been made where necessary to contact holders of copyright to obtain permission to reproduce copyright material. If any have been inadvertently overlooked, the publisher will be pleased to make the necessary arrangements at the first opportunity. The **CD/DVD-ROM** (if any) provided in the sealed envelope with this book is complimentary and free of cost. **Not meant for sale.**

Inquiries for bulk sales may be solicited at: jaypee@jaypeebrothers.com

Color Atlas of Dermatophytoses: Focus on Superficial Fungal Infections / *Jayakar Thomas, Parimalam Kumar*

First Edition: **2021**

ISBN: 978-93-89188-38-7

Dedicated to

The many dermatologists who provide care to their patients with dermatophytoses, our committed teachers of Dermatology, the patients who were willing to permit us to take their photographs and most of all to our beloved spouses for their care, love and affection without which this humble piece of work would not have been a reality.

FOREWORD

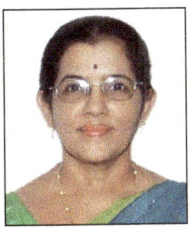

UR Dhanalakshmi MD DD DNB

Former Professor and Head
Department of Dermatology
Madras Medical College
Chennai, Tamil Nadu, India

It is a privilege to write the foreword for the book edited by Professor Jayakar Thomas. I have listened to numerous orations and talks delivered by him as well as gone through a lot of his books, chapters in books and articles.

In medicine, it is important to diagnose and treat common conditions more effectively rather than concentrating on rare disorders since the bulk of our patients fall into the former category.

Dermatophytoses are one of the commonest conditions encountered in clinical practice and it is also one of the most psychologically crippling disorders. The social and psychological aspects of acne are very important notably because it affects individuals during adolescence when personality development takes place. Above all, the scourge today is the development of drug resistance, added on by the indiscriminate use of topical steroids.

Therefore it is important to hit dermatophytoses early and hit it hard. It is also important to rule out various conditions associated with dermatophytoses.

Color Atlas of Dermatophytoses: Focus on Superficial Fungal Infections cover every aspect of this group of diseases and should be read by every dermatologist since the bulk of patients coming to a dermatologist have this problem. The images and legends are especially informative and help in easy understanding.

I congratulate the co-editor Dr Parimalam Kumar for working alongside Dr Jayakar Thomas in compiling this book. I also convey my best wishes to them in coming up with similar work in the future.

PREFACE

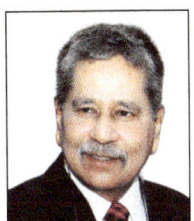

Jayakar Thomas
MD DD MNAMS FRCP FRCPCH PhD DSc
Professor and Head
Department of Dermatology
Sree Balaji Medical College and Hospital
Chennai, Tamil Nadu, India

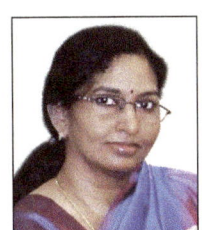

Parimalam Kumar
MD DD MNAMS FRCP
Professor and Head
Department of Dermatology
Stanley Medical College and Hospital
Chennai, Tamil Nadu, India

"Knowledge, if not shared is of no use at all"

Dermatophytoses are amongst one of the most common skin condition worldwide. Despite this fact, accurate information about this condition is scarce.

This book, *Color Atlas of Dermatophytoses: Focus on Superficial Fungal Infections*, is designed as an academic project with the target readers as both postgraduate students and practicing dermatologist. All chapters encompass glimpses of existing knowledge in the light of recent advances in the segment of fungal diseases and the comorbidities. We are duty-bound to thank our residents Dr Sivaramakrishnan Sangaiah and Dr Shreya Srinivasan who helped us capture some of the photographs.

We hope this book is a helpful tool, not only for the student who needs an expert source of basic knowledge in the different forms of dermatophytoses, but also for the pressured practitioner who needs a clear, concise, and balanced distillation of the best information on which to base daily clinical decisions.

At times, the science presented might seem overwhelming to the reader. But one can start reading from any chapter, based on one's interests, tastes, and preferences.

Jayakar Thomas
Parimalam Kumar

CONTENTS

1. Scalp Infections — 1
2. Face Infections — 11
3. Trunk and Limbs Infection — 26
4. Axillary Infections — 85
5. Hand Infections — 89
6. Groin Infections — 98
7. Gluteal Area Infections — 127
8. Feet Infections — 147
9. Nail Infections — 152
10. Steroid-modified Disease — 157
11. Infections in Pregnancy — 176
12. Infections in Children — 184
13. Infections in Adolescent — 209
14. Infections in the Immunocompromised — 227
15. Mimickers of Dermatophytoses — 245

CHAPTER 1
Scalp Infections

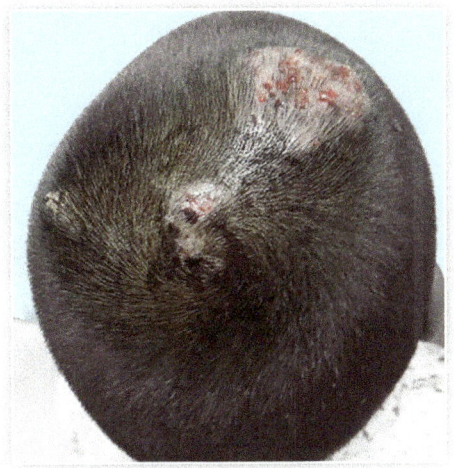

FIG. 1: Kerion note the boggy swellings.

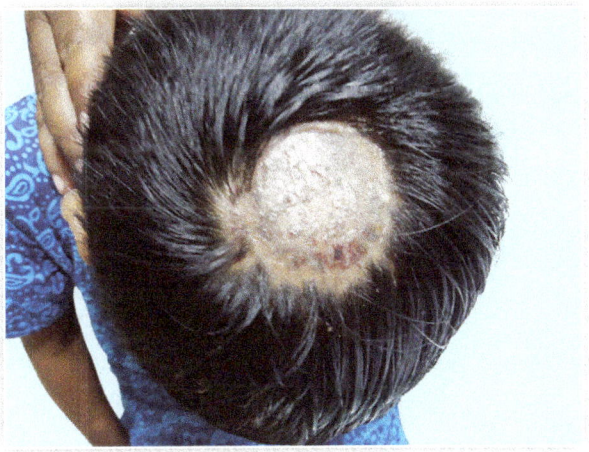

FIG. 2: Boggy swelling misinterpreted as abscess and treated with antibiotic usage.

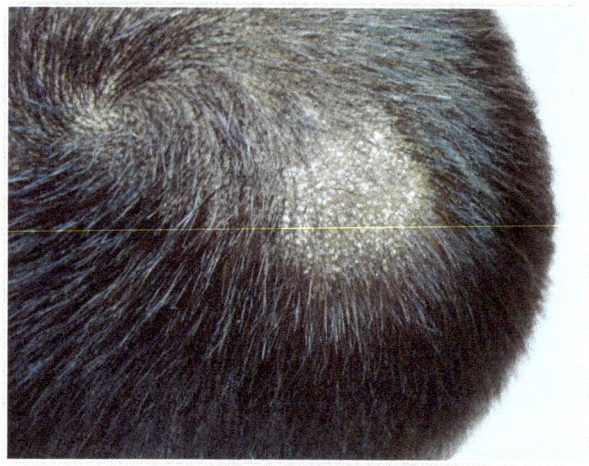

FIG. 3: Gray-patch type of tinea capitis.

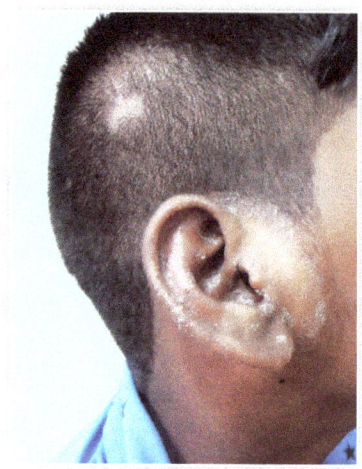

FIG. 4: Alopecia areata type of tinea capitis, note the involvement of the pinna.

Scalp Infections

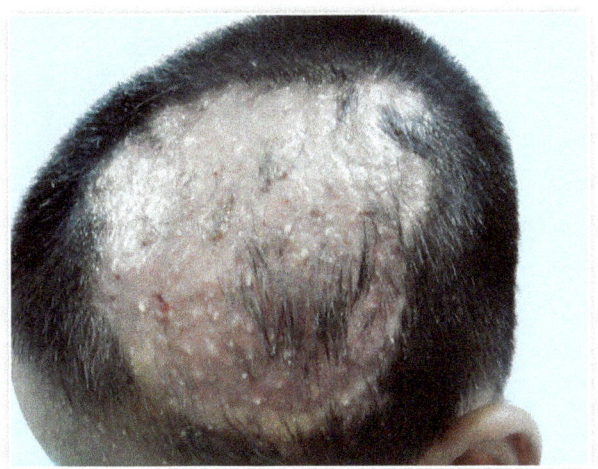

FIG. 5: Multiple pustules in a child with tinea capitis.

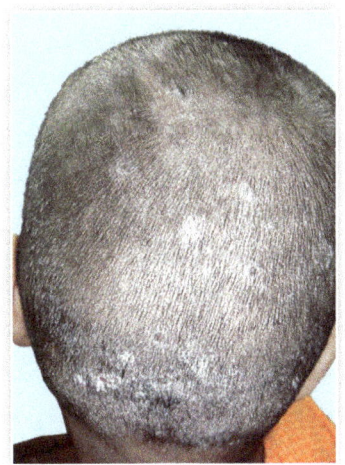

FIG. 6: Noninflammatory type of tinea capitis in a child.

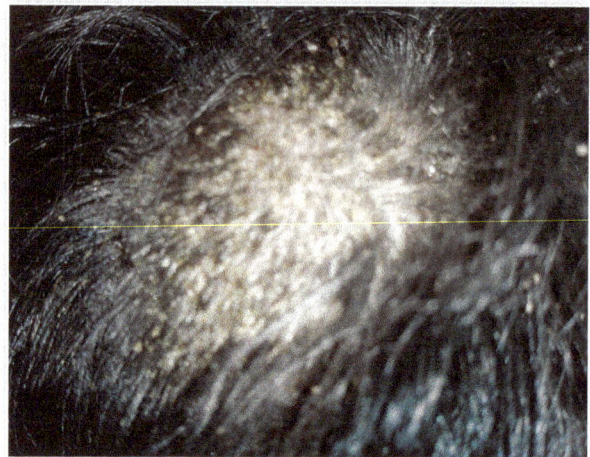

FIG. 7: Tinea capitis with intense scaling.

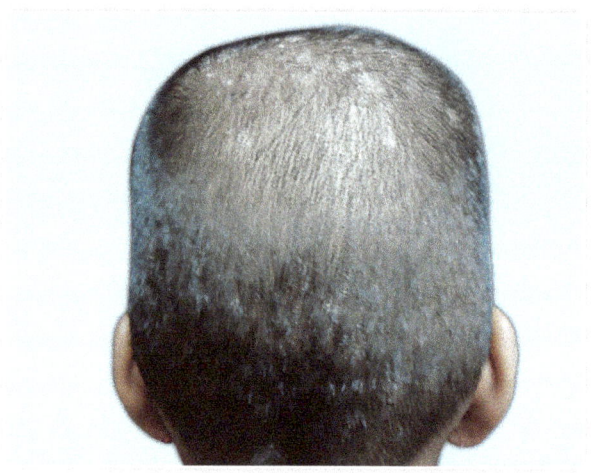

FIG. 8: Noninflammatory gray patch type of tinea capitis.

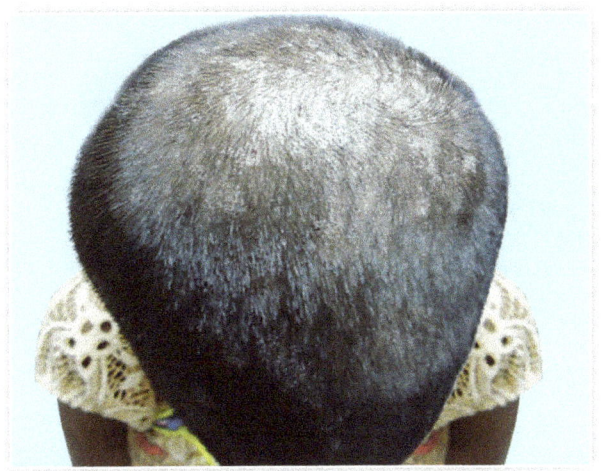

FIG. 9: Same patient as in figure 8.

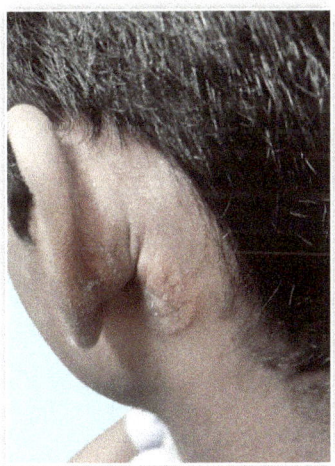

FIG. 10: Glabrous type of tinea capitis.

Color Atlas of Dermatophytoses: *Focus on Superficial Fungal Infections*

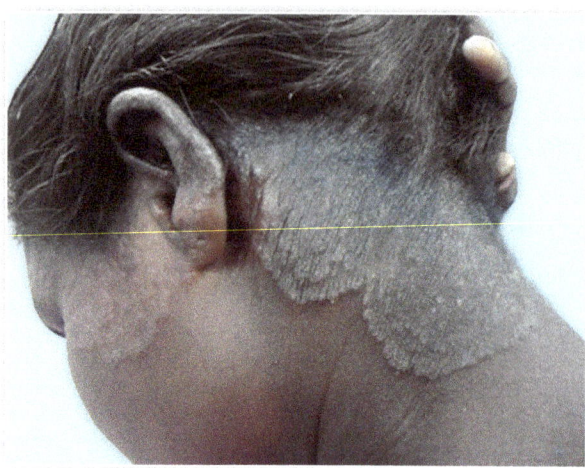

FIG. 11: Glabrous type of tinea capitis in an adult. Note extension on to the face.

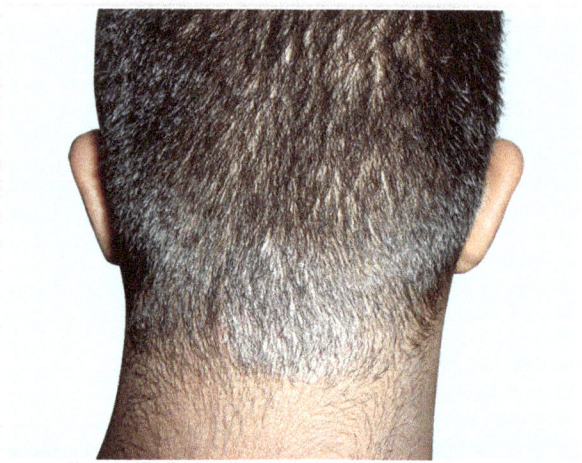

FIG. 12: Tinea capitis in an adult mimicking psoriasis.

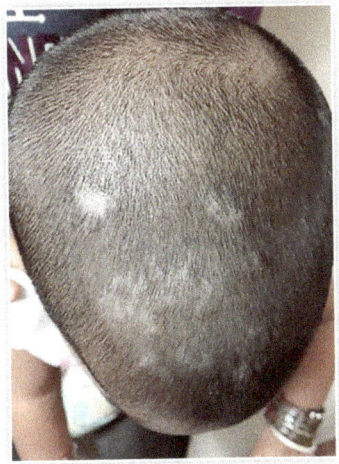

FIG. 13: Multiple patches of tinea capitis well seen after tonsuring.

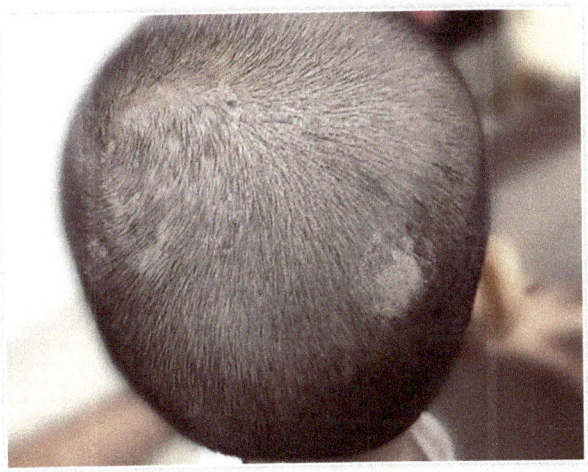

FIG. 14: Same patient as in figure 13.

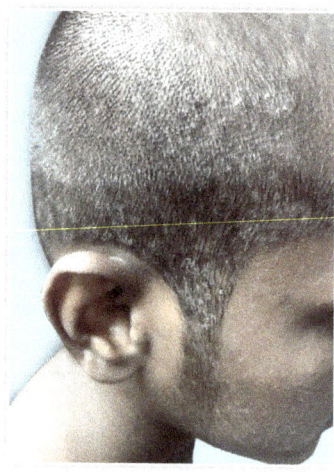

FIG. 15: Glabrous type of tinea capitis. Note the involvement of face.

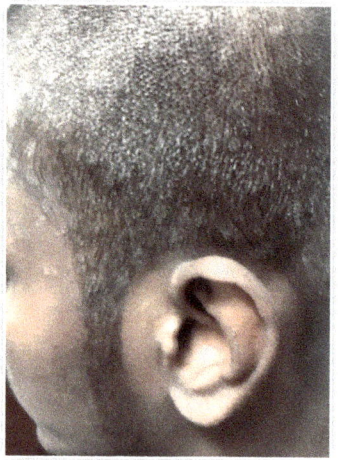

FIG. 16: Same patient as in figure 15.

Scalp Infections

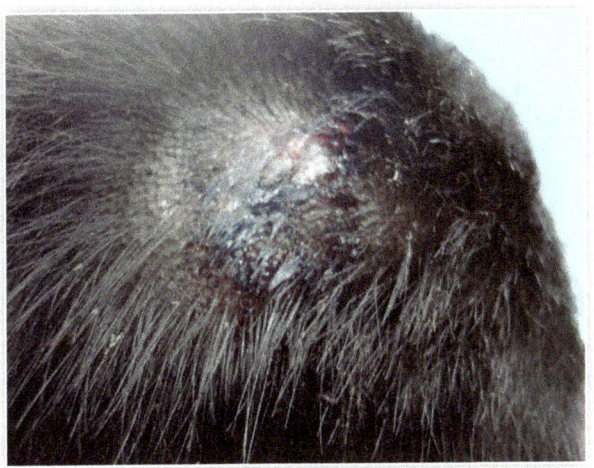

FIG. 17: Kerion with secondary bacterial infection.

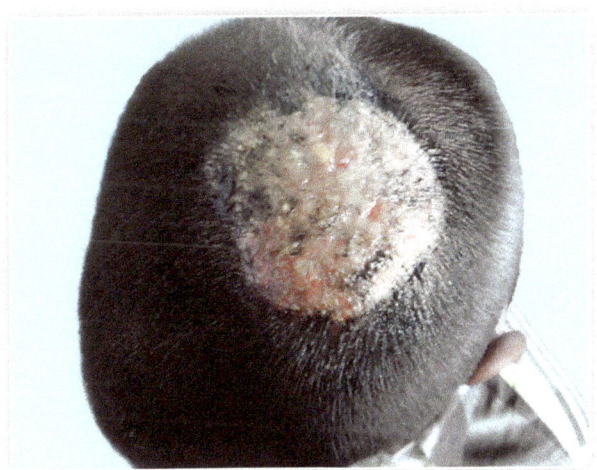

FIG. 18: Kerion and inflammatory type of tinea capitis.

Color Atlas of Dermatophytoses: *Focus on Superficial Fungal Infections*

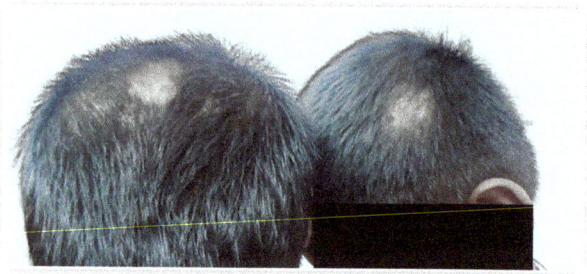

FIG. 19: Tinea capitis in brothers.

Face Infections

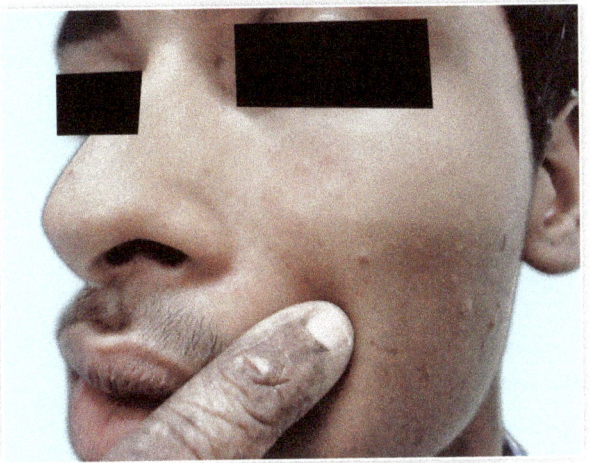

FIG. 1: Tinea faciei around the left eye. This might involve the eye lashes and needs prolonged treatment.

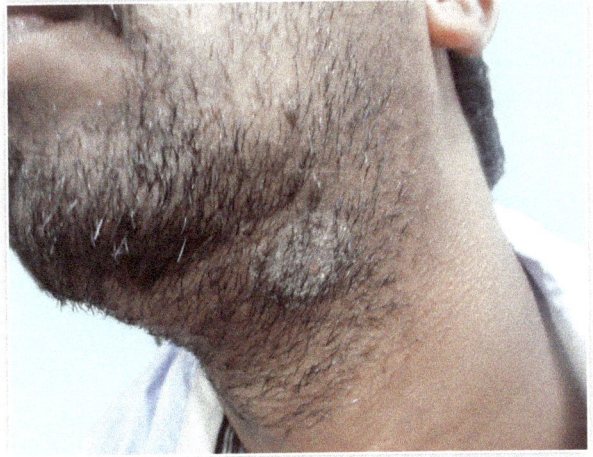

FIG. 2: Single patch involving the beard area.

Color Atlas of Dermatophytoses: *Focus on Superficial Fungal Infections*

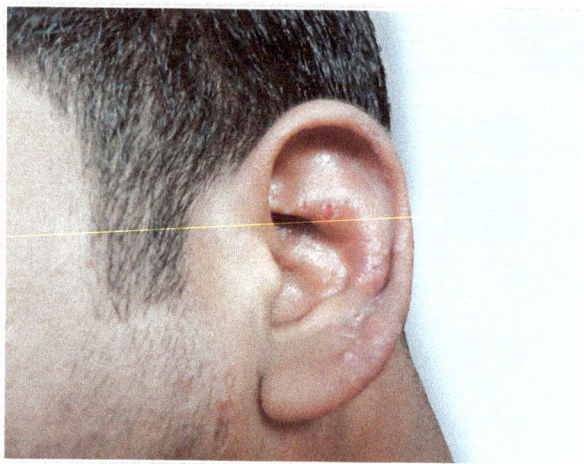

FIG. 3: Involvement of pinna with excoriation.

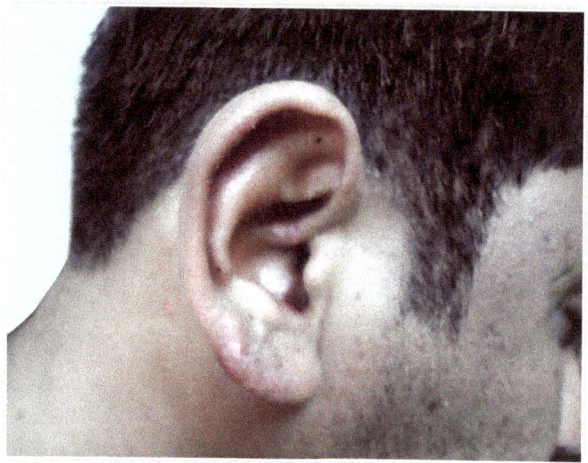

FIG. 4: Same patient as in figure 3 indicating autoinfection.

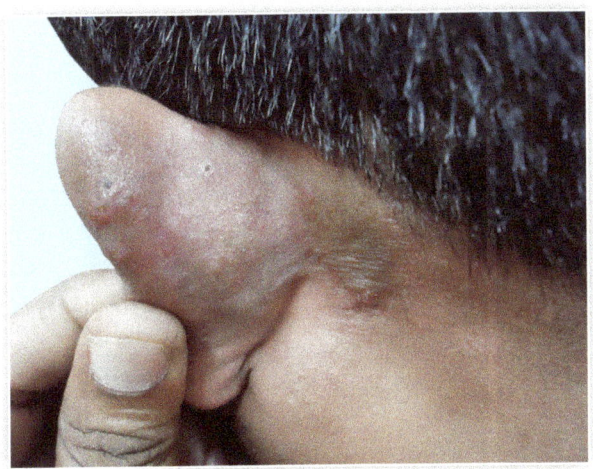

FIG. 5: Retroauricular involvement.

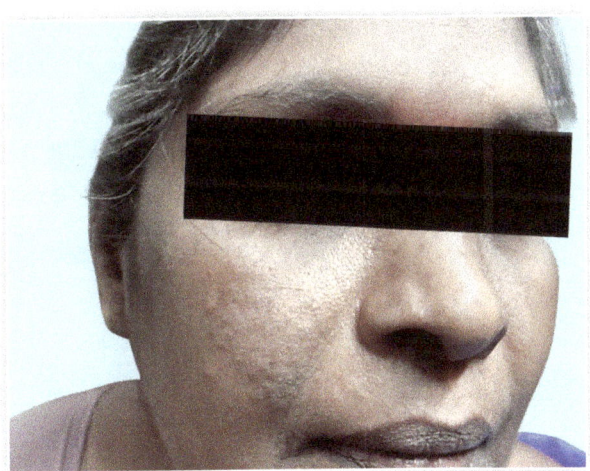

FIG. 6: Noninflammatory type of tinea faciei.

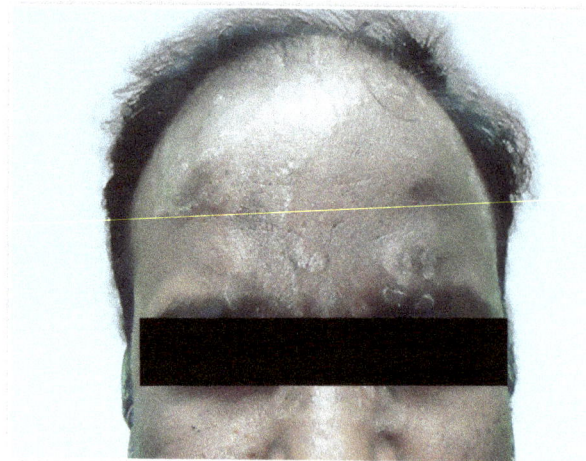

FIG. 7: Extensive tinea faciei extending on to the bald scalp.

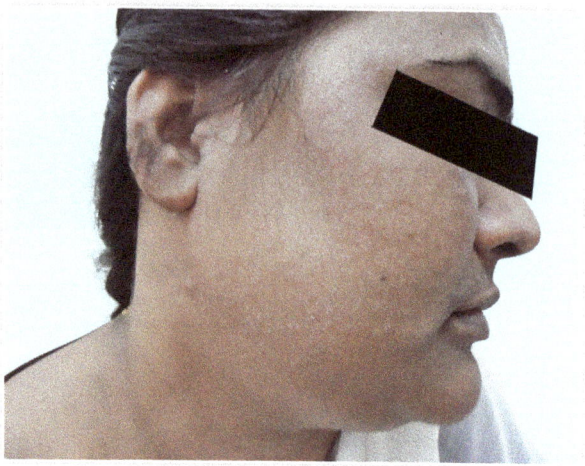

FIG. 8: Tinea faciei with very mild scaling.

Face Infections

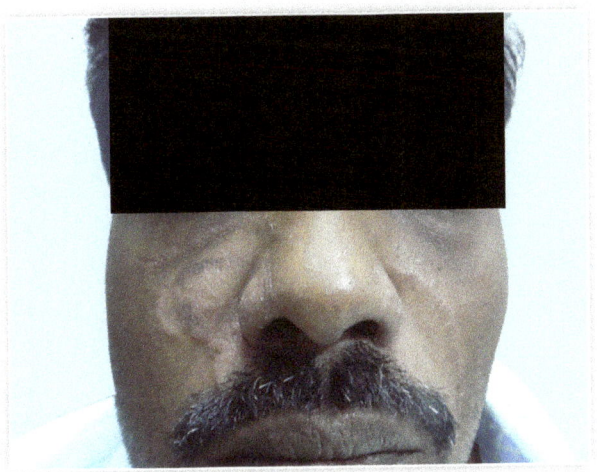

FIG. 9: Involvement of midface. Note the well-defined border.

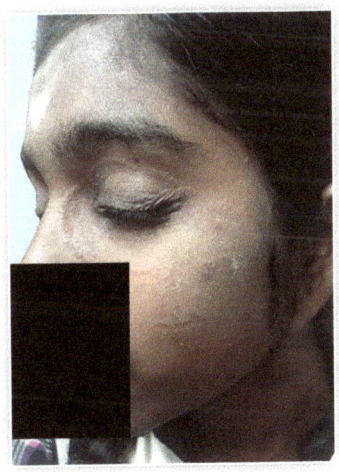

FIG. 10: Involvement of periorbital area will need systemic antifungal therapy.

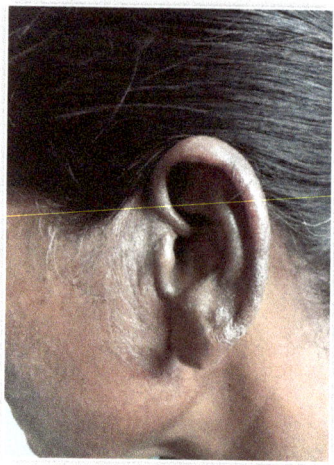

FIG. 11: Tinea faciei unilateral involvement of the ear, a diagnostic clue.

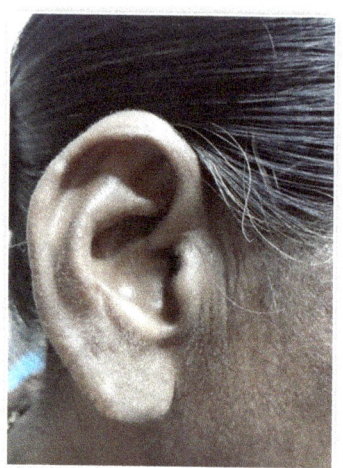

FIG. 12: Same patient as in figure 11. Note there is no involvement of the right side.

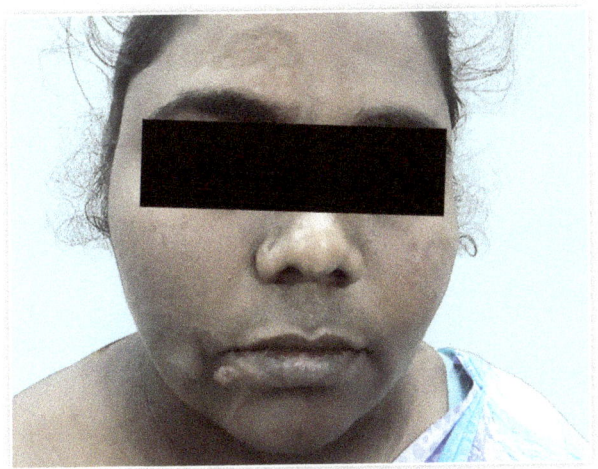

FIG. 13: Tinea faciei treated with topical steroid, note herpes simplex.

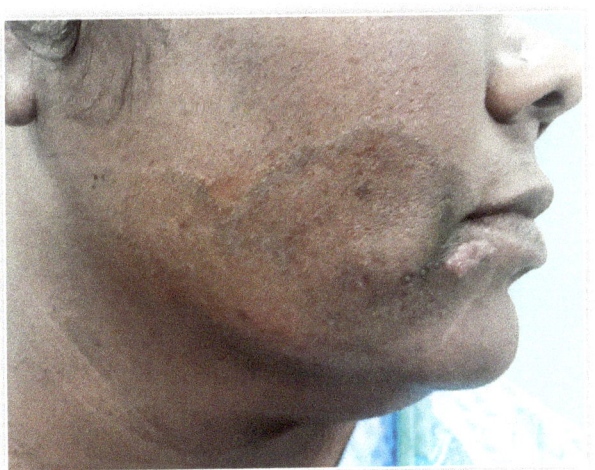

FIG. 14: Same patient as in figure 13. Note the well-defined border over the right cheek.

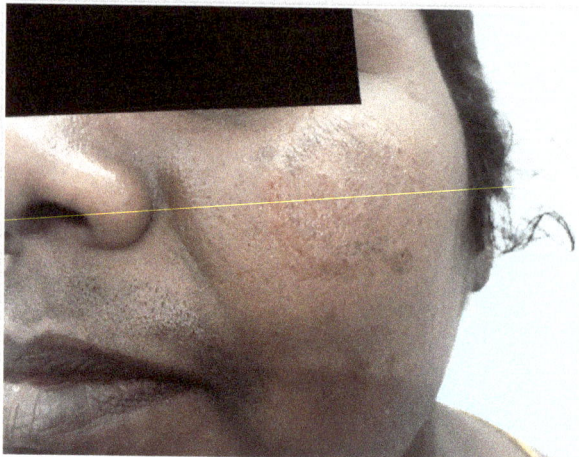

FIG. 15: Same patient as in figures 13 and 14 involvement of left side of face.

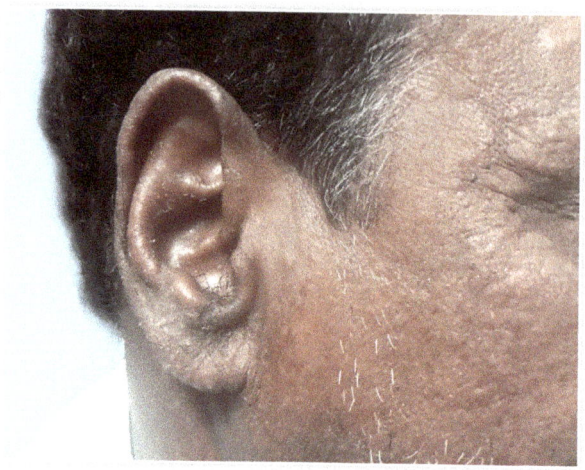

FIG. 16: Very faint scaling in a patient with tinea faciei.

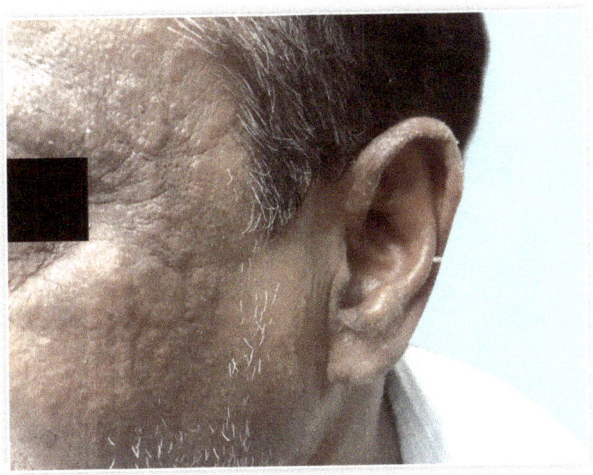

FIG. 17: Same patient as in figure 16. Note border in the preauricular area.

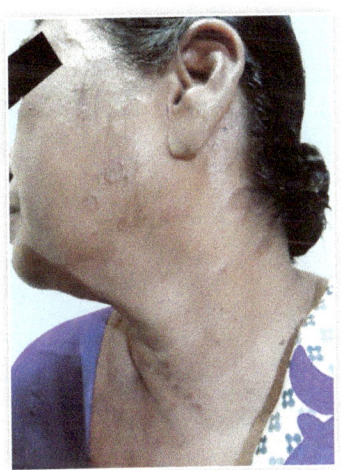

FIG. 18: Tinea faciei in a patient with psoriasis.

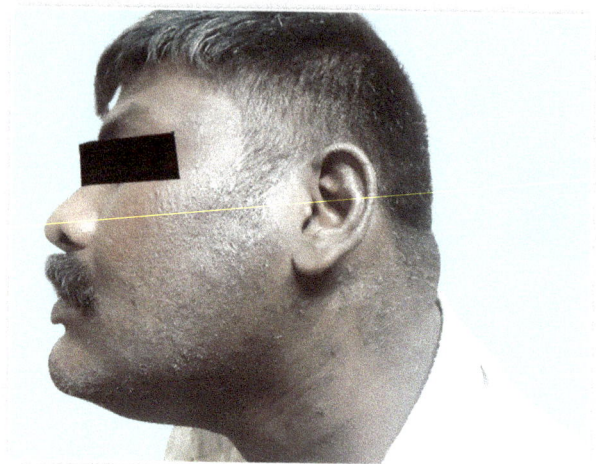

FIG. 19: Ill-defined scaly patch.

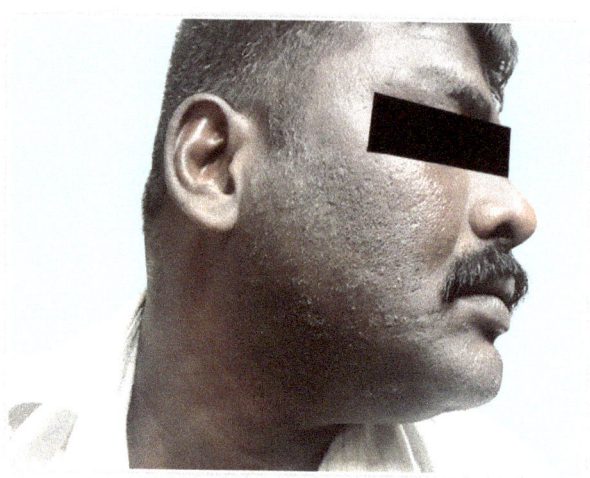

FIG. 20: Same patient as in figure 19 showing patches over the neck as well.

Face Infections

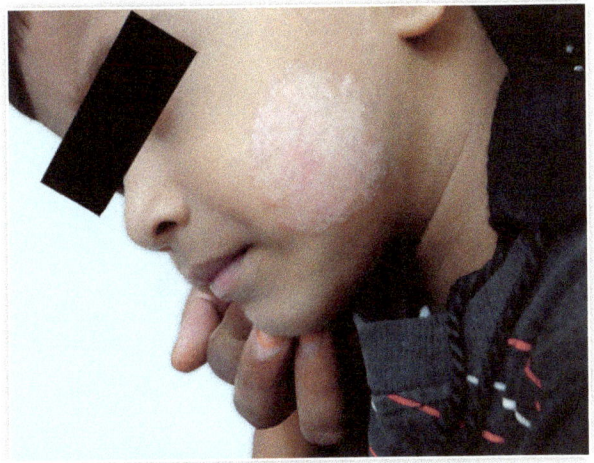

FIG. 21: Tinea faciei in a boy whose father also had tinea faciei.

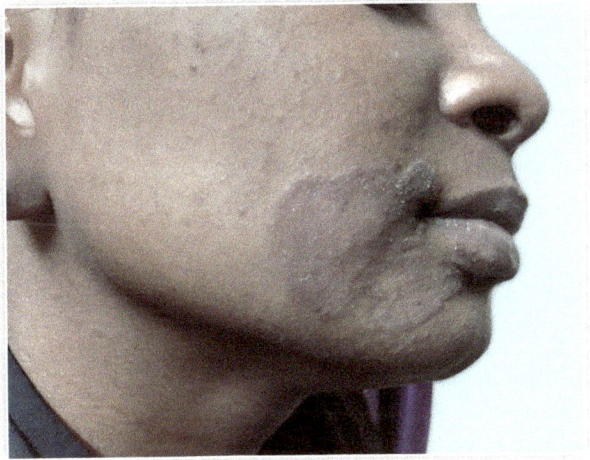

FIG. 22: Involvement of the vermilion border in tinea faciei.

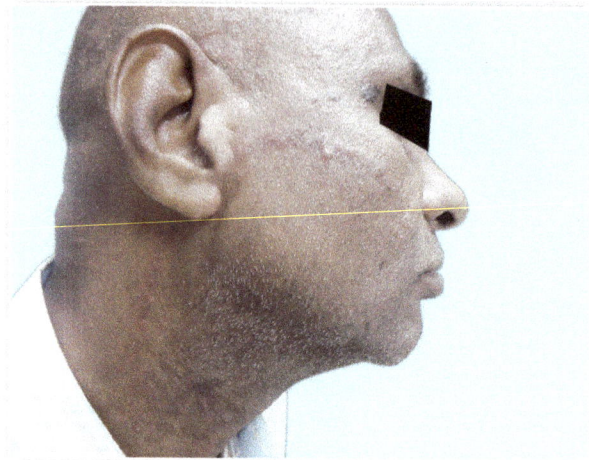

FIG. 23: The active border without much scaling in a man with tinea faciei.

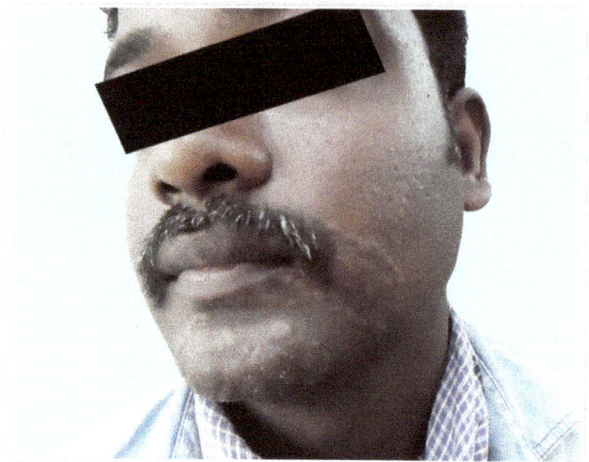

FIG. 24: Patch within patch affecting the perioral area.

Face Infections

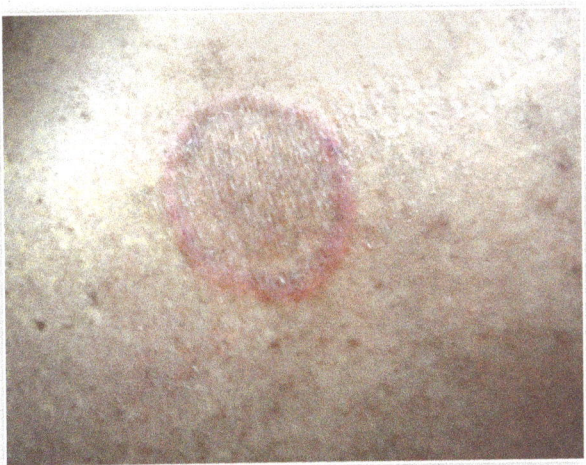

FIG. 25: Single coin shaped tinea faciei; centre showing inflammation.

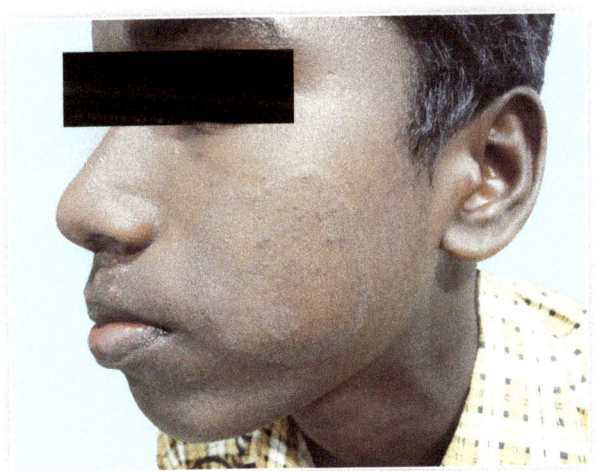

FIG. 26: Small patch within a big patch of tinea faciei.

Color Atlas of Dermatophytoses: *Focus on Superficial Fungal Infections*

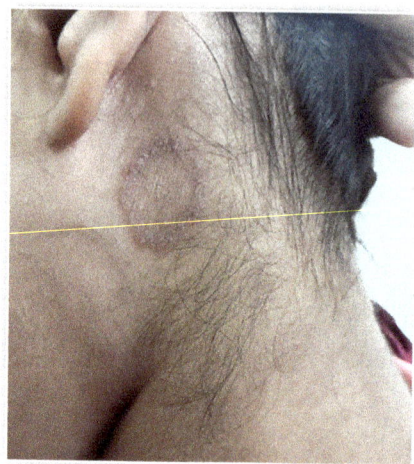

FIG. 27: Classical annular scaly patch involving the neck.

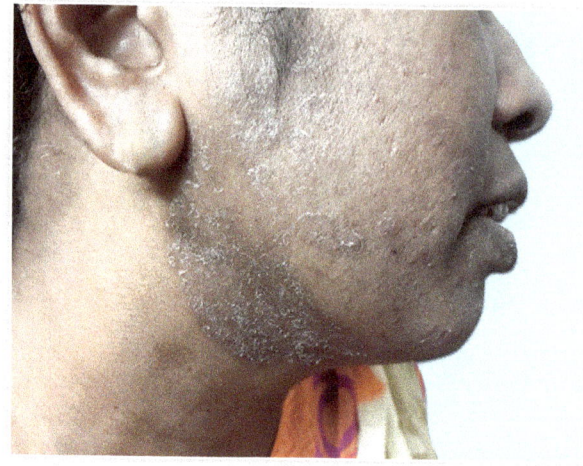

FIG. 28: Extensive scaling yet asymptomatic in a noninflammatory type.

Face Infections

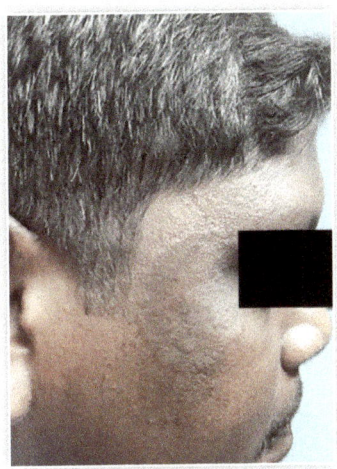

FIG. 29: Ill-defined border difficulty in diagnosis in dark individuals.

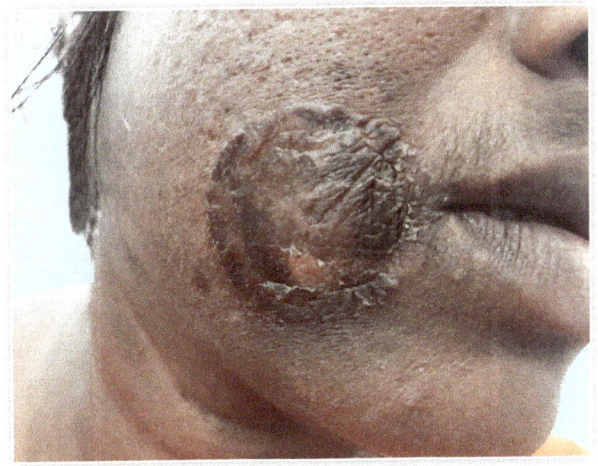

FIG. 30: Tinea faciei worsened with topical steroid.

CHAPTER 3: Trunk and Limbs Infection

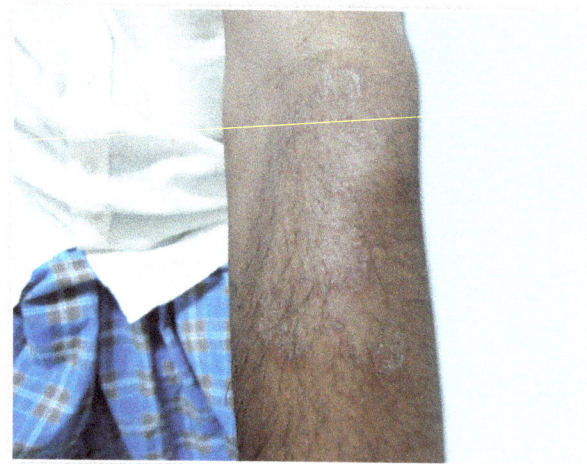

FIG. 1: Tinea corporis affecting the arm.

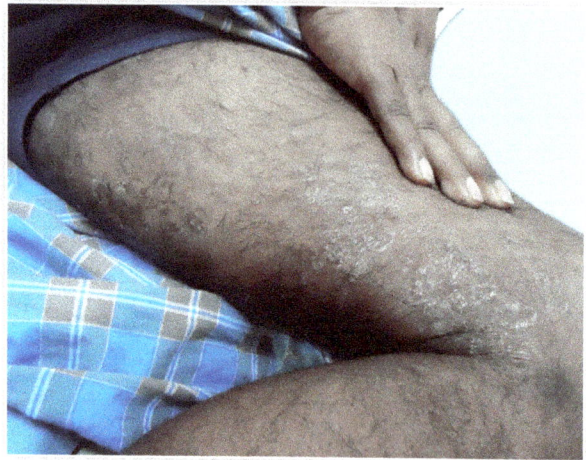

FIG. 2: Same patient as in figure 1 showing involvement of the thigh.

Trunk and Limbs Infection

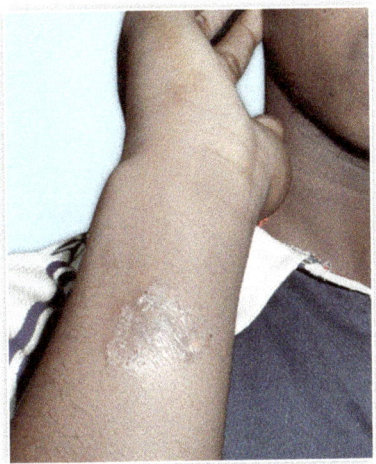

FIG. 3: Tinea corporis in a painter mistaken for eczema.

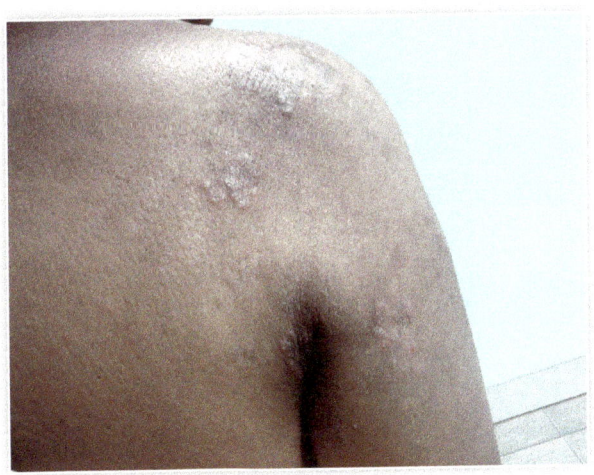

FIG. 4: Multiple patches of tinea corporis.

Color Atlas of Dermatophytoses: *Focus on Superficial Fungal Infections*

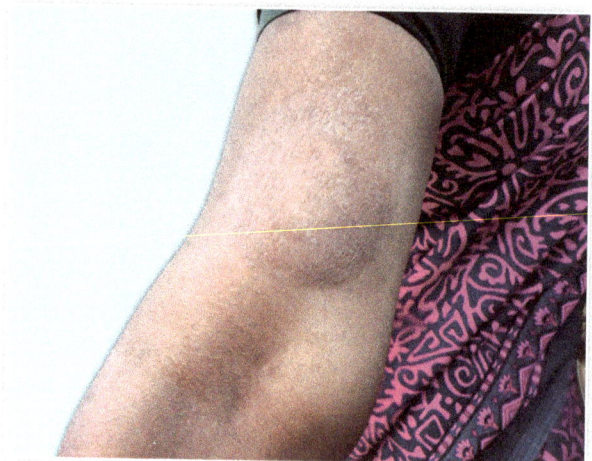

FIG. 5: Ill-defined border of tinea corporis following treatment.

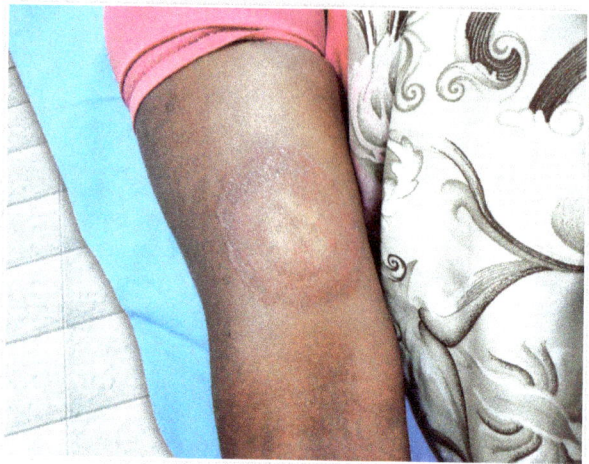

FIG. 6: Classical annular patch with central clearance.

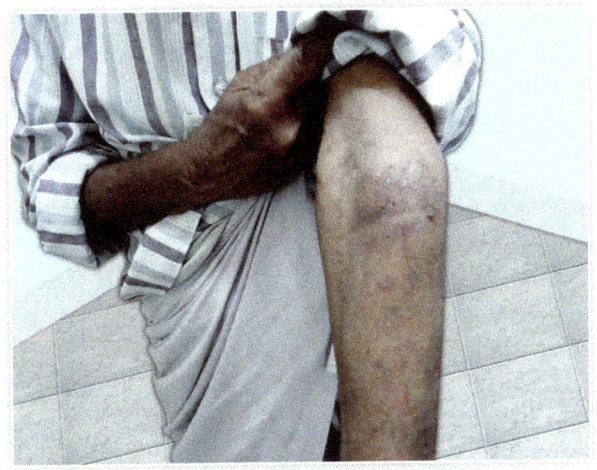

FIG. 7: Inflammatory type of tinea corporis in an elderly man.

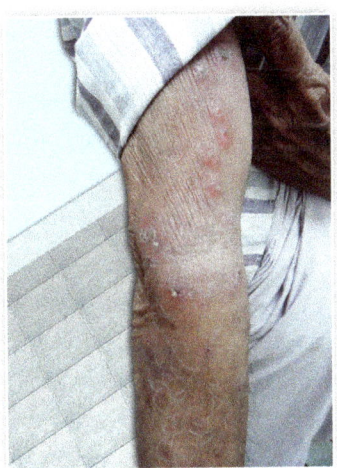

FIG. 8: Same patient as in figure 7.

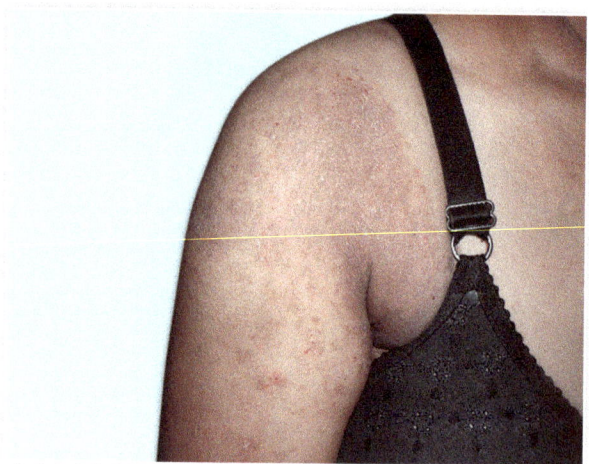

FIG. 9: Shoulder involvement in a woman.

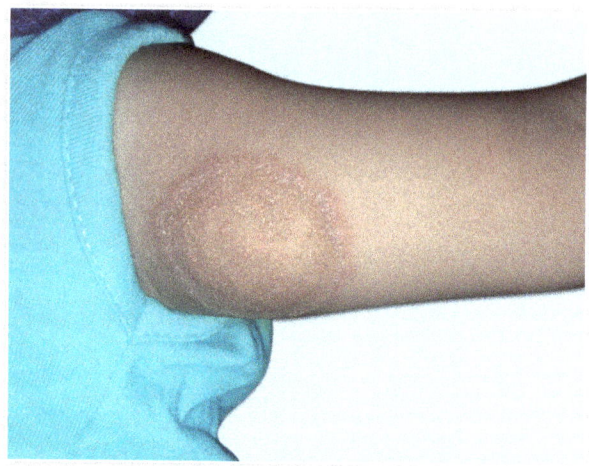

FIG. 10: Classical well-defined annular patch with active border.

Trunk and Limbs Infection

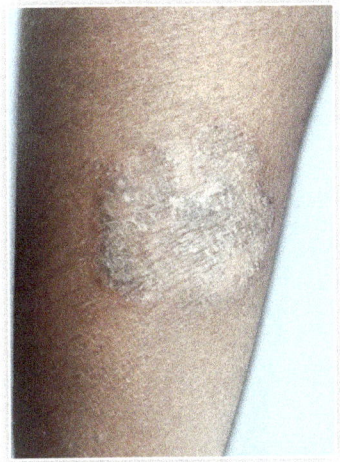

FIG. 11: Ill-defined border in partially treated case.

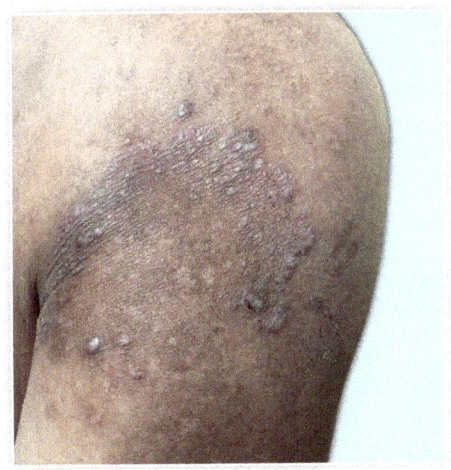

FIG. 12: Border active in one end and ill-defined at the other.

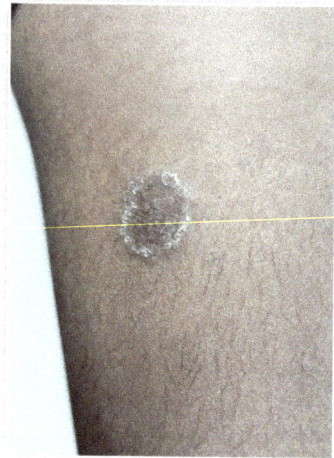

FIG. 13: Single patch with active margin.

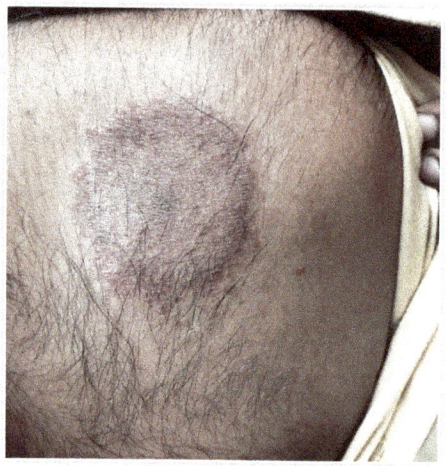

FIG. 14: Resistant patch of tinea after two months of treatment.

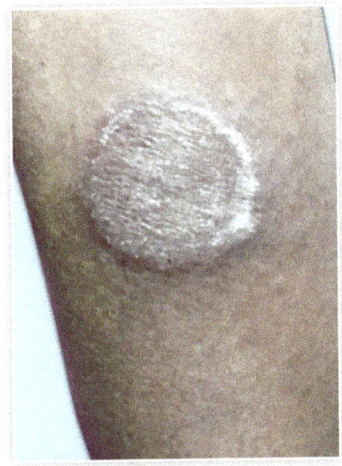

FIG. 15: Asymptomatic patch treated as psoriasis with topical steroid.

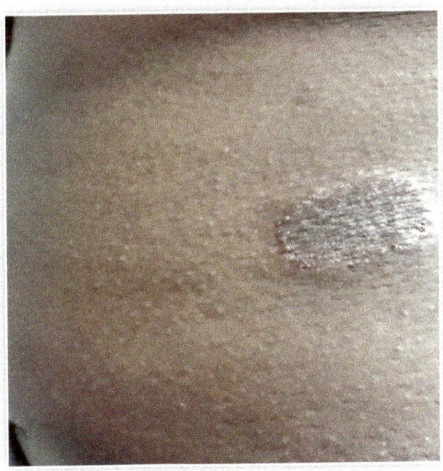

FIG. 16: Well-defined small patch.

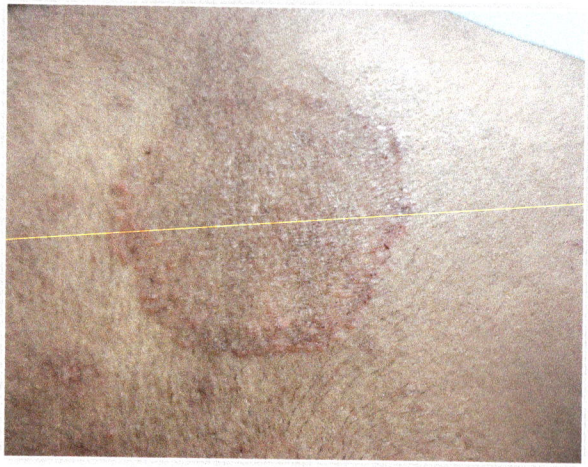

FIG. 17: Erythema and scaling indicating active infection.

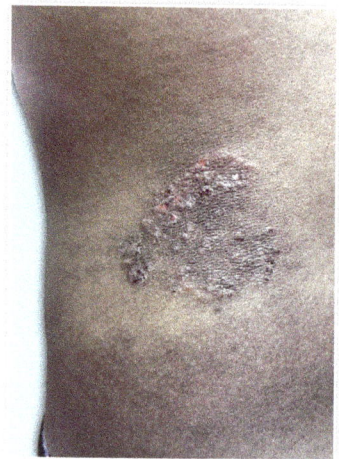

FIG. 18: Inflammatory type showing excoriation marks.

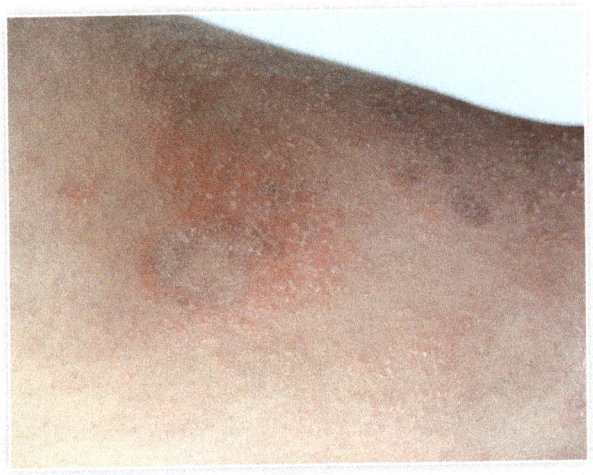

FIG. 19: Intense erythema and pustules posing diagnostic difficulty.

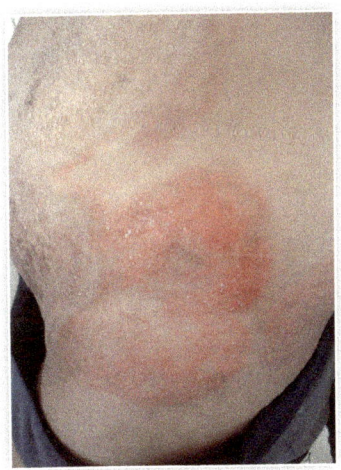

FIG. 20: Same patient as in figure 19 with a better delineated morphology.

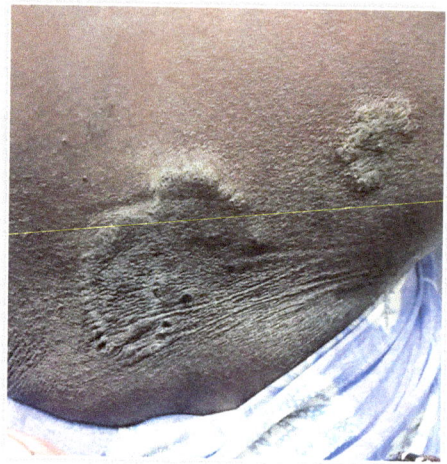

FIG. 21: Annular and arciform plaques of tinea corporis.

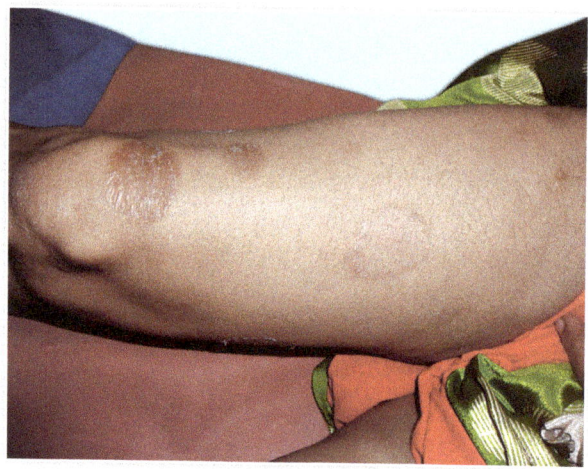

FIG. 22: Healed as well as the active patch.

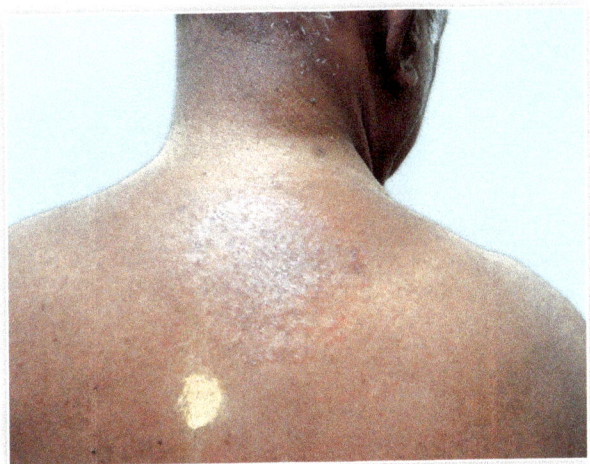

FIG. 23: Single ill-defined patch with slight scaling.

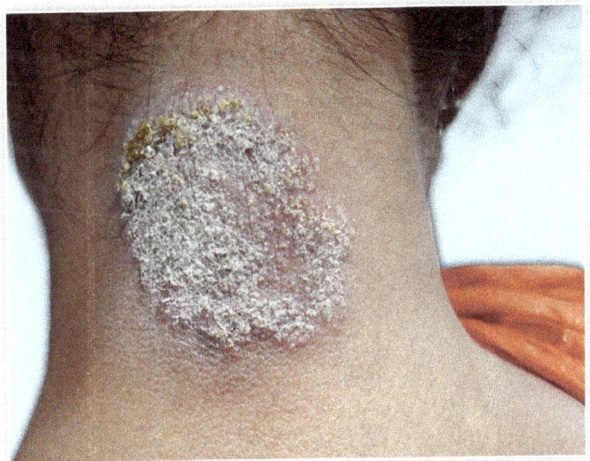

FIG. 24: Inflammatory type of tinea corporis.

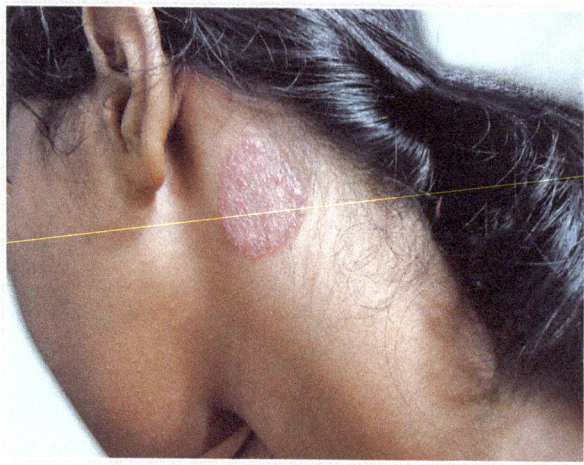

FIG. 25: Inflammatory type of tinea corporis mimicking psoriasis.

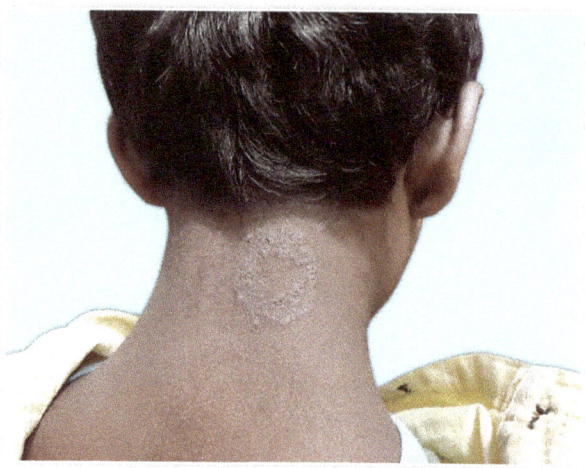

FIG. 26: Classical morphology of annular patch.

Trunk and Limbs Infection

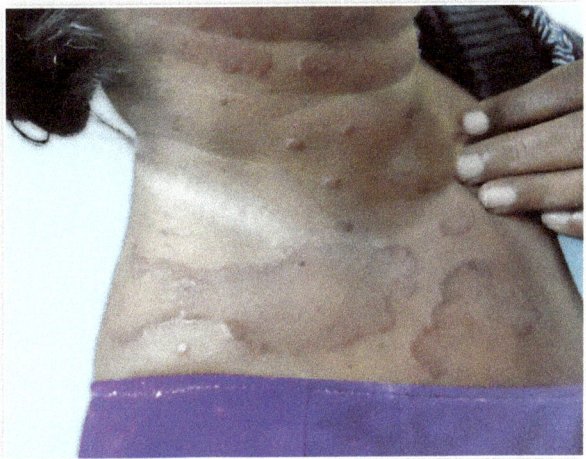

FIG. 27: Acriform patches involving the shoulder and chest.

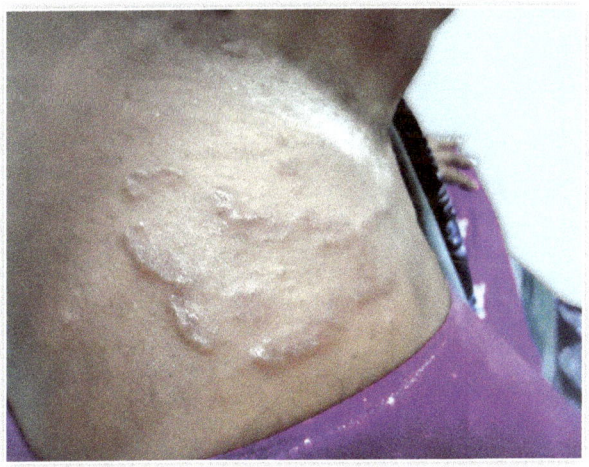

FIG. 28: Same patient as figure 27 showing the well defined margin.

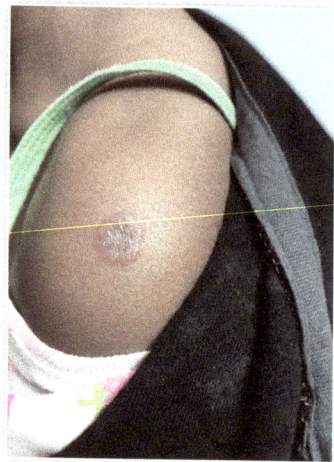

FIG. 29: Early lesion of tinea corporis.

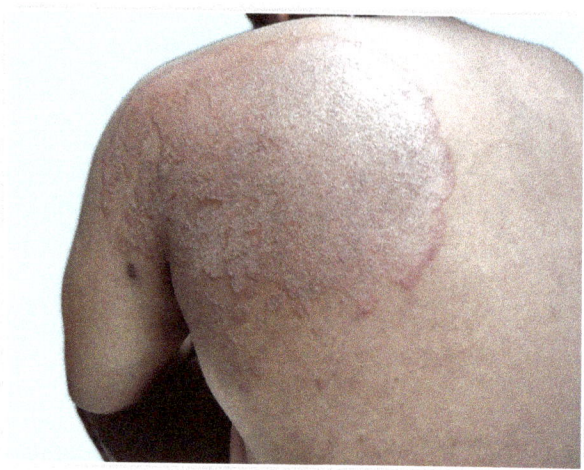

FIG. 30: Asymptomatic patch of tinea corporis.

Trunk and Limbs Infection

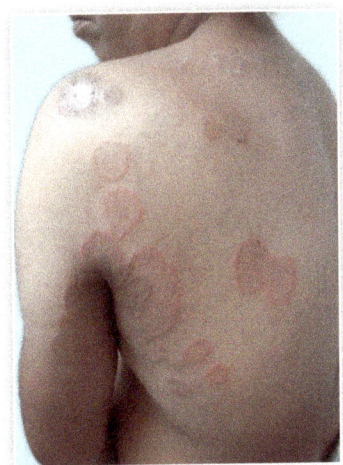

FIG. 31: Extensive tinea corporis.

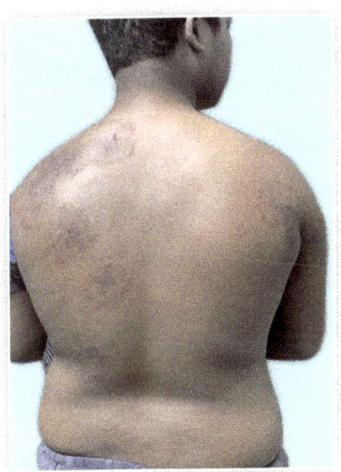

FIG. 32: Multiple patches in a man on long-term systemic steroids.

Color Atlas of Dermatophytoses: *Focus on Superficial Fungal Infections*

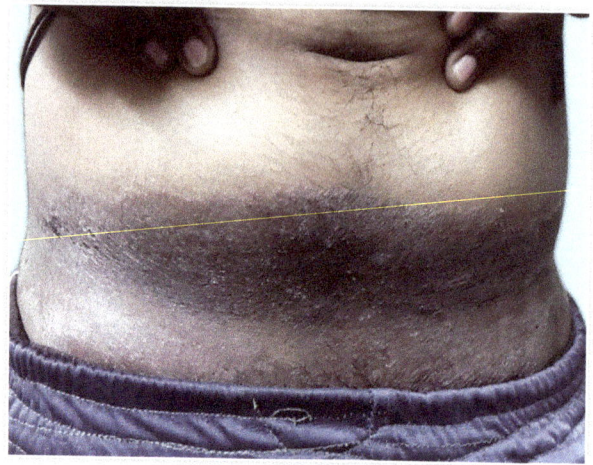

FIG. 33: Entire waist area being involved with scaly margin.

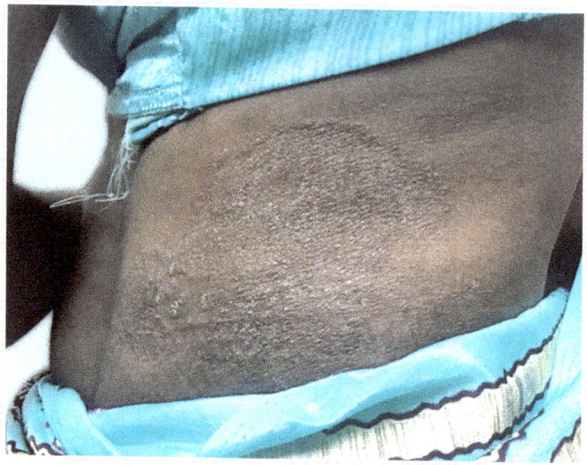

FIG. 34: Asymptomatic noninflammatory type.

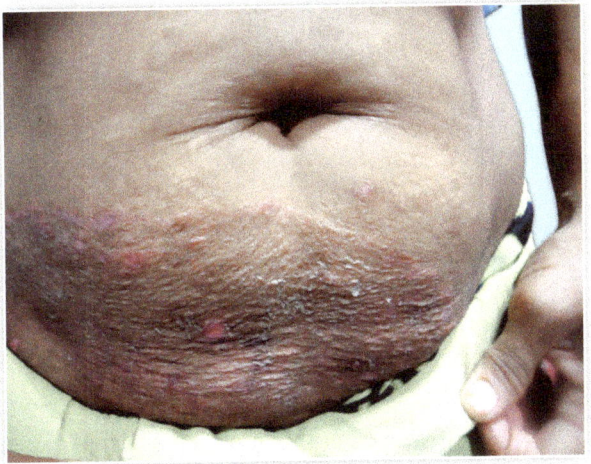

FIG. 35: Tinea corporis with scaling and erosion.

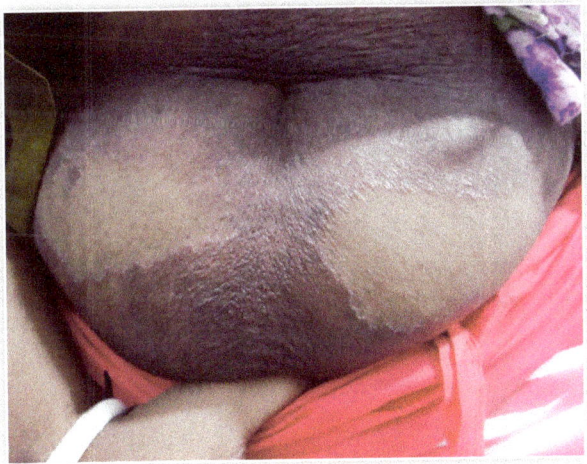

FIG. 36: Extensive tinea corporis with islands of normal skin.

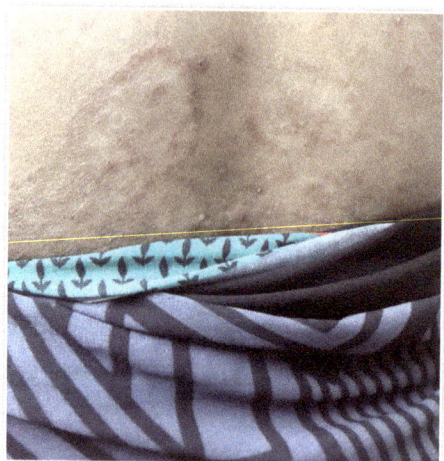

FIG. 37: Tinea corporis showing healing active margin.

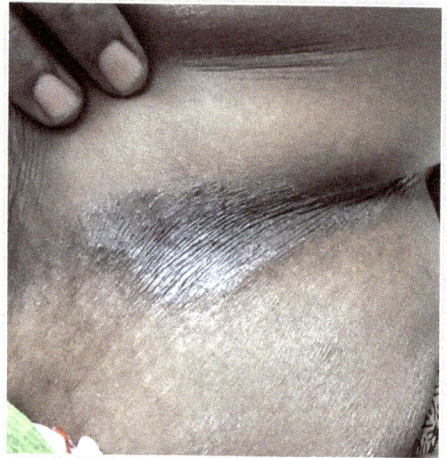

FIG. 38: Tinea corporis over intertriginous fold.

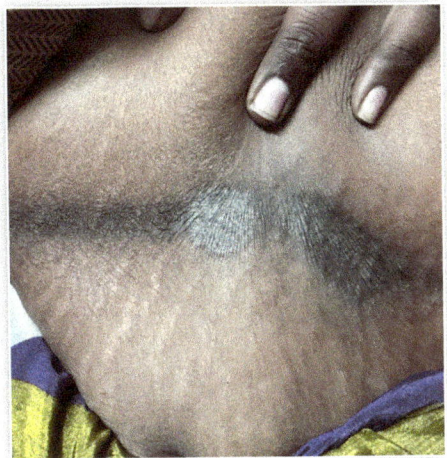

FIG. 39: Same patient as in figure 38.

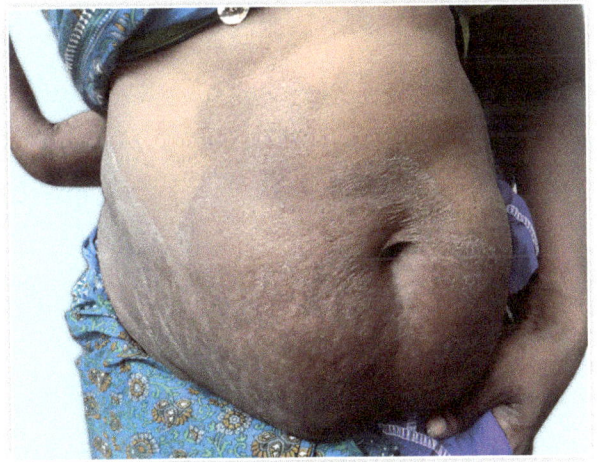

FIG. 40: Extensive tinea corporis.

Color Atlas of Dermatophytoses: *Focus on Superficial Fungal Infections*

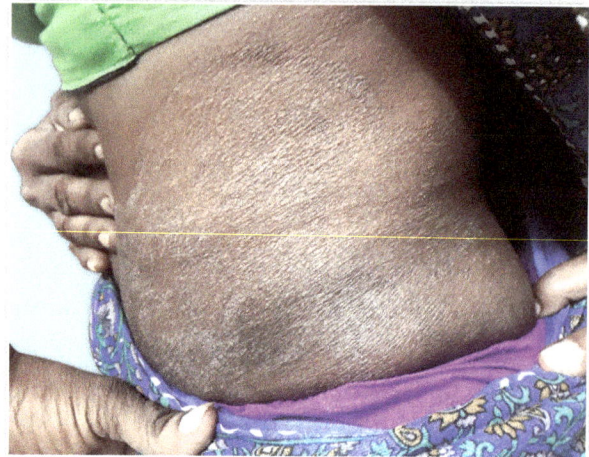

FIG. 41: Same patient as in figure 40.

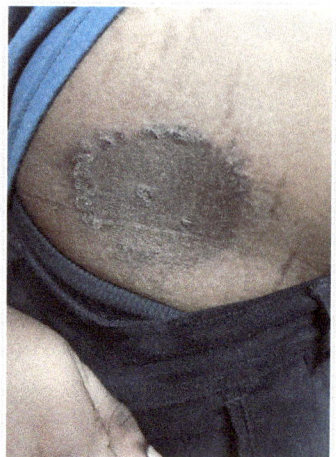

FIG. 42: Single patch, with well-defined margin.

Trunk and Limbs Infection

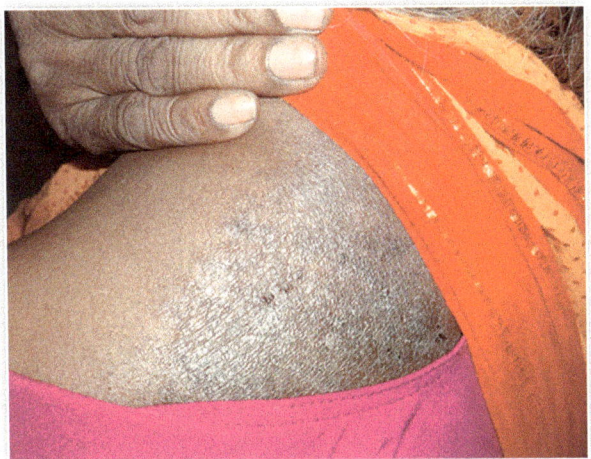

FIG. 43: Sweating and occlusion common precipitating factor.

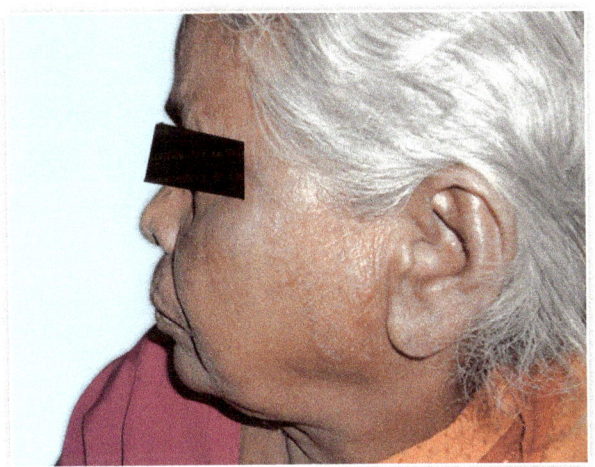

FIG. 44: Same patient as in figure 43.

Color Atlas of Dermatophytoses: *Focus on Superficial Fungal Infections*

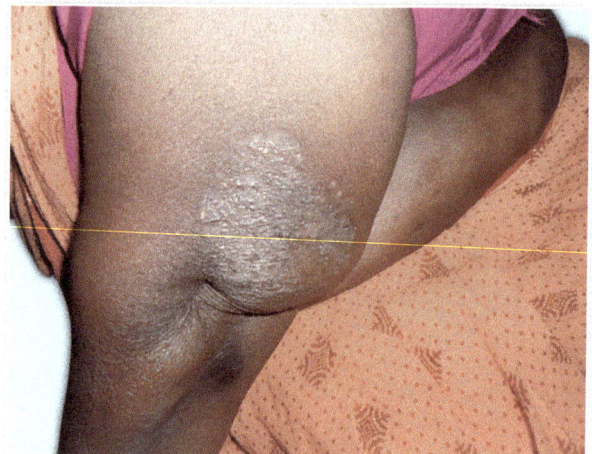

FIG. 45: Same patient as in figure 44.

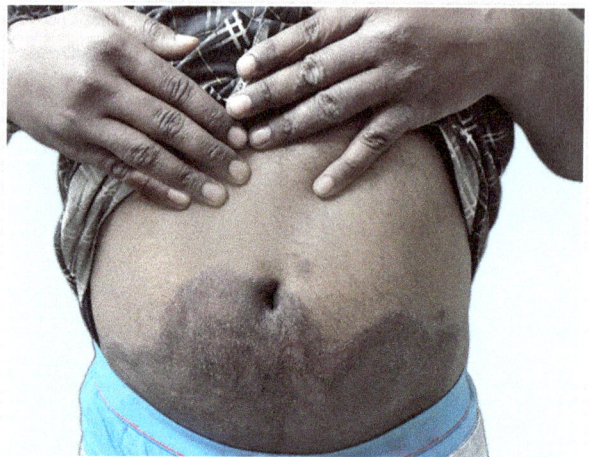

FIG. 46: Extensive involvement in an obese male.

Trunk and Limbs Infection

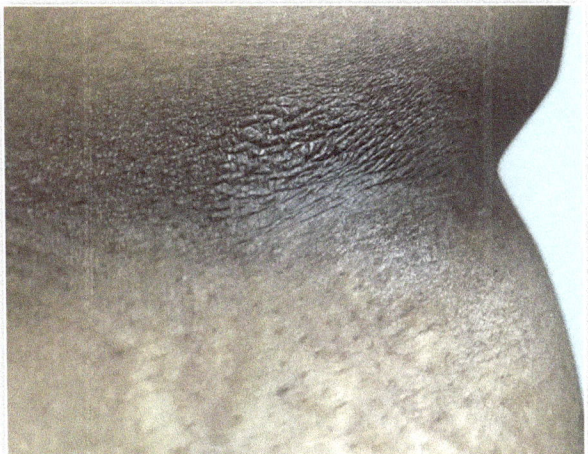

FIG. 47: Tinea corporis taking lichenoid appearance.

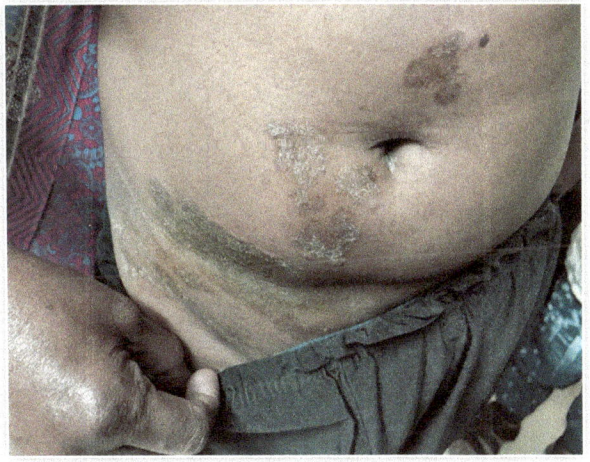

FIG. 48: Tinea corporis with scaly irregular patches.

Color Atlas of Dermatophytoses: *Focus on Superficial Fungal Infections*

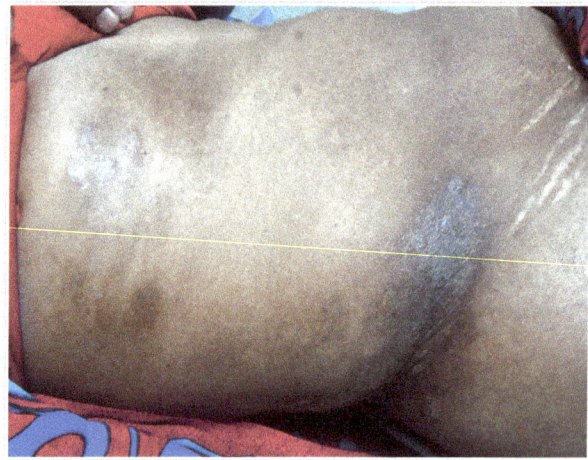

FIG. 49: Frictional keratosis with small patches of tinea corporis.

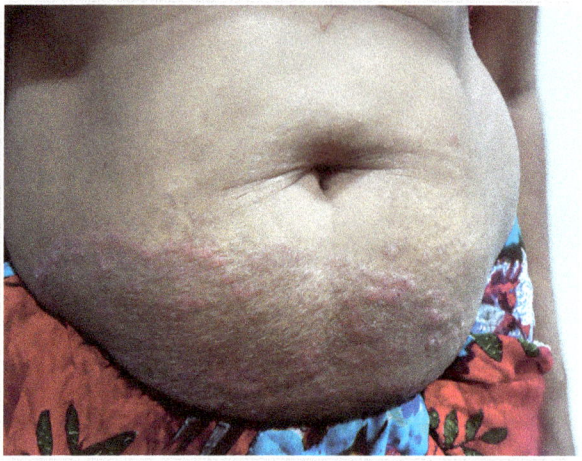

FIG. 50: Same patient as in figure 49 having classical tinea corporis.

Trunk and Limbs Infection

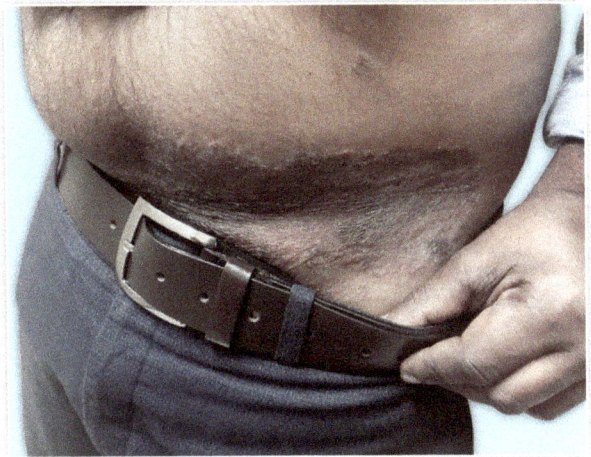

FIG. 51: Tinea corporis. Note the tight occlusive clothing.

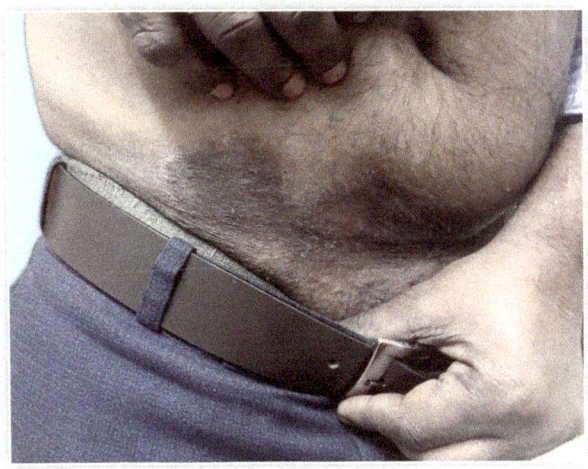

FIG. 52: Same patient as in figure 51.

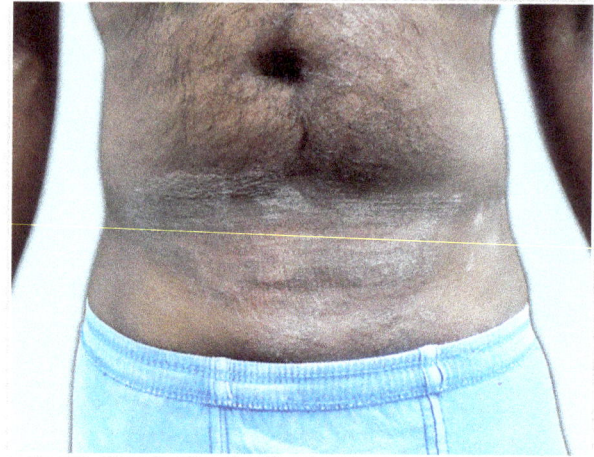

FIG. 53: Large patch affecting lower abdomen.

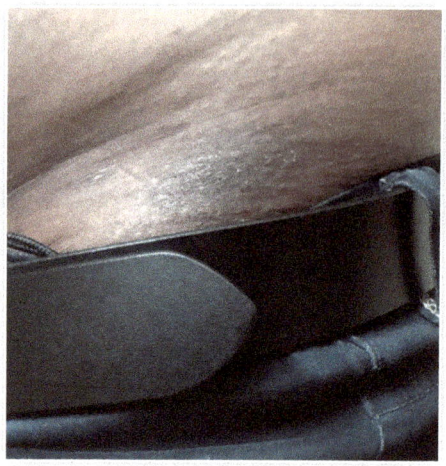

FIG. 54: The margin give to the clue to diagnosis of tinea corporis.

Trunk and Limbs Infection

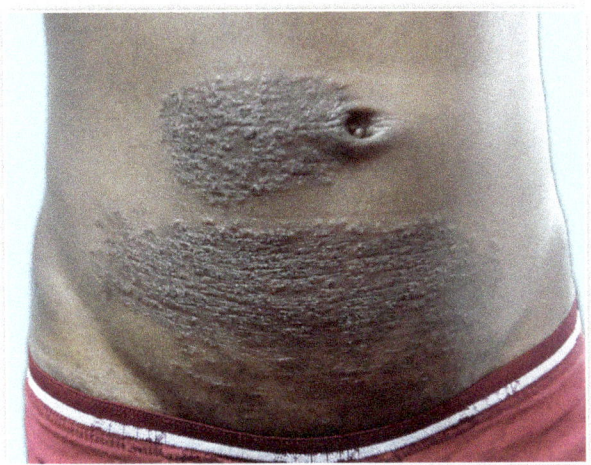

FIG. 55: The pigmentation and small papules set over the patch.

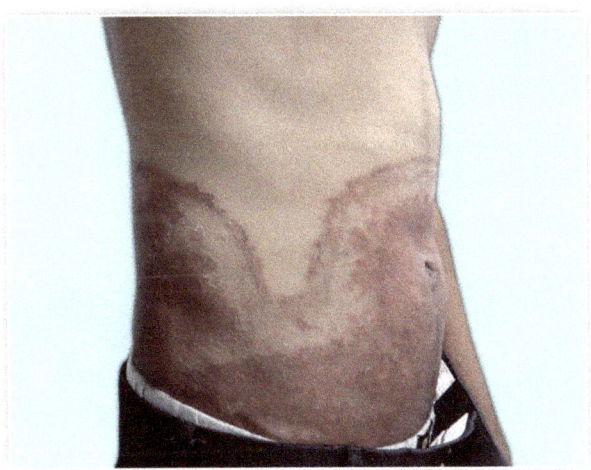

FIG. 56: Extensive tinea corporis.

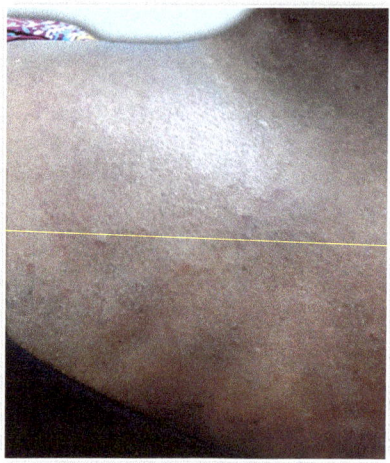

FIG. 57: Partially treated tinea corporis.

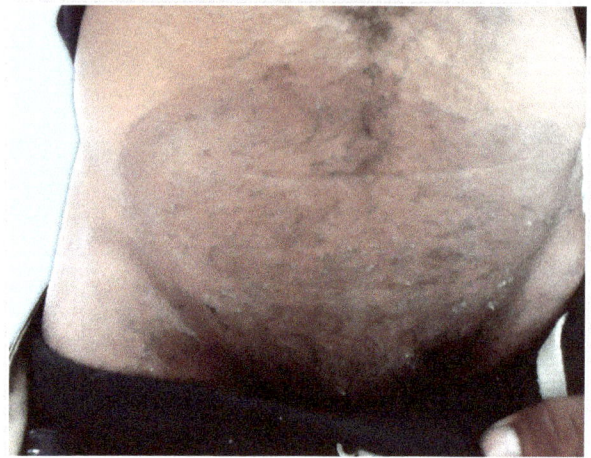

FIG. 58: Noninflammatory tinea corporis with minimal scaling.

Trunk and Limbs Infection

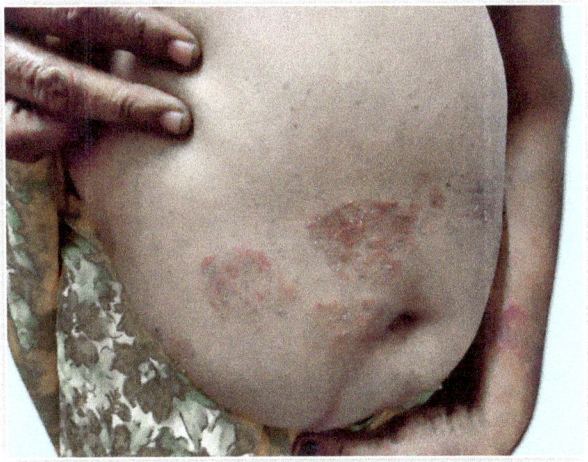

FIG. 59: Multiple patches. Note involvement of the forearm.

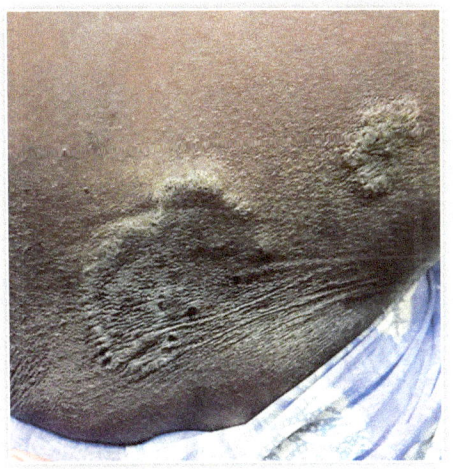

FIG. 60: Multiple annular patches of tinea corporis.

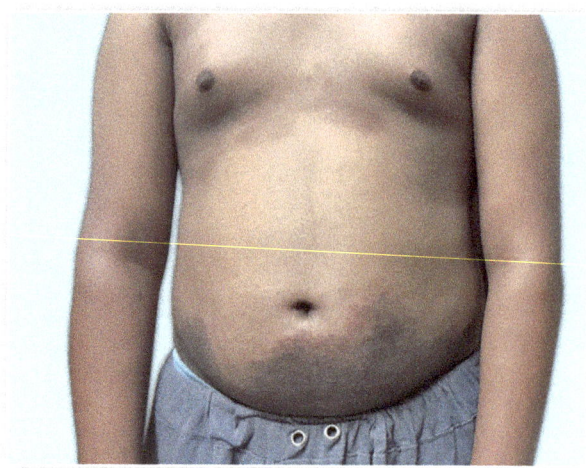

FIG. 61: Tinea corporis.

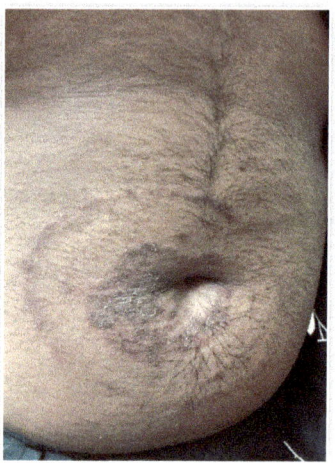

FIG. 62: Concentric rings over the periumbilical area.

Trunk and Limbs Infection

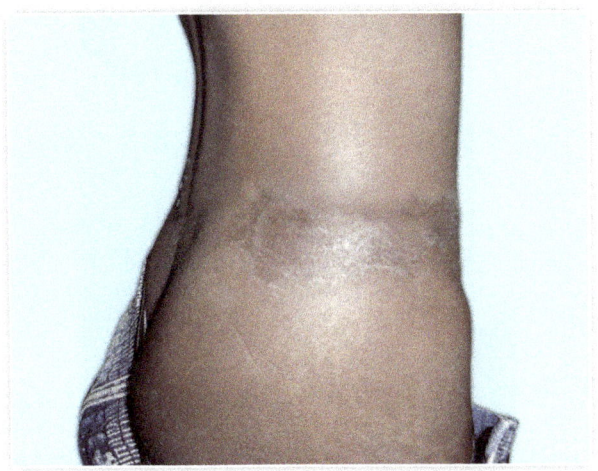

FIG. 63: Waist string is a common source of reinfection.

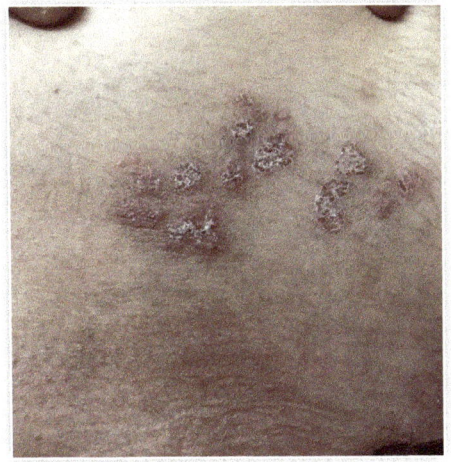

FIG. 64: Psoriasiform scales.

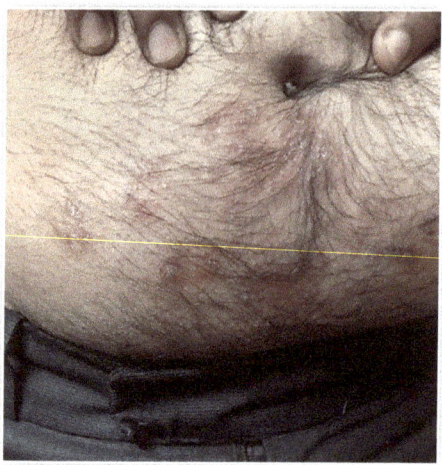

FIG. 65: Ill-defined scaly patches.

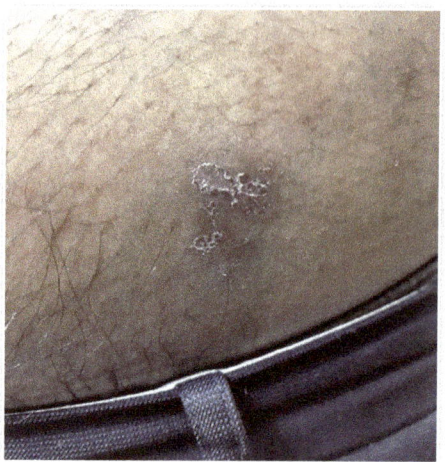

FIG. 66: Same patient as in figure 65.

Trunk and Limbs Infection

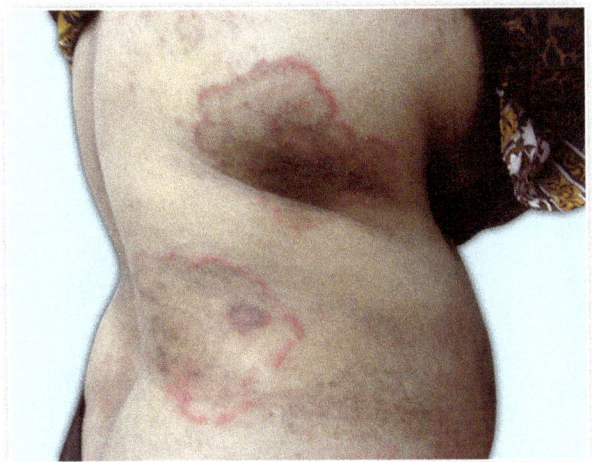

FIG. 67: Multiple well-defined patches of tinea corporis.

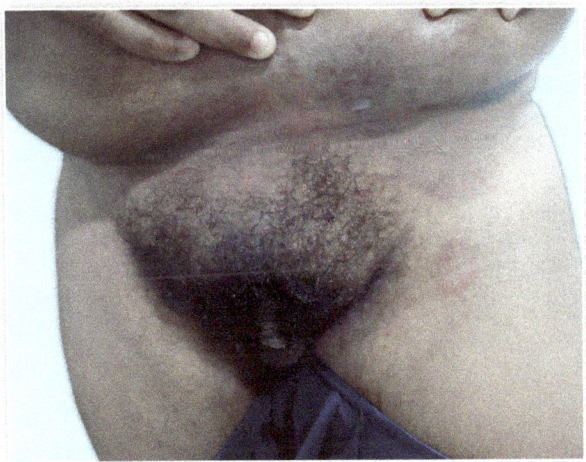

FIG. 68: Tinea corporis also involving the genital.

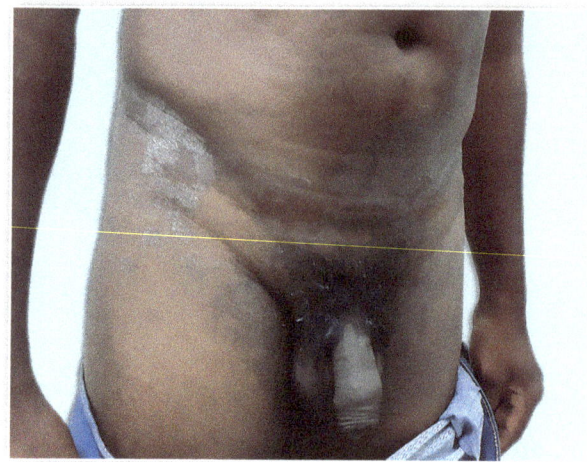

FIG. 69: Tinea corporis - the waist cord is always a source of reinfection.

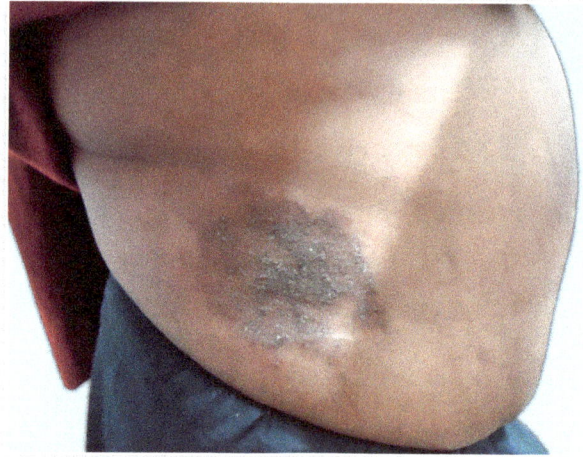

FIG. 70: Irregular patch of tinea corporis with scaling.

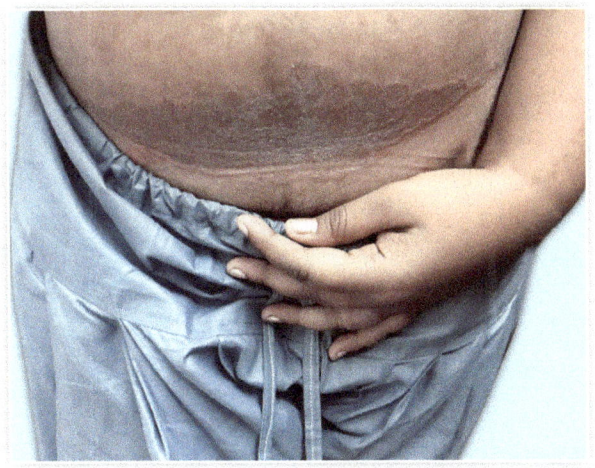

FIG. 71: Tinea corporis of the waist with well-defined margin.

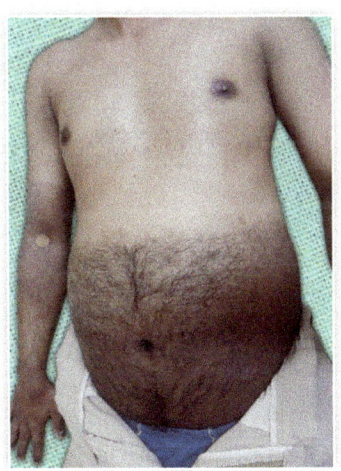

FIG. 72: Ill-defined large scaly patch of tinea corporis.

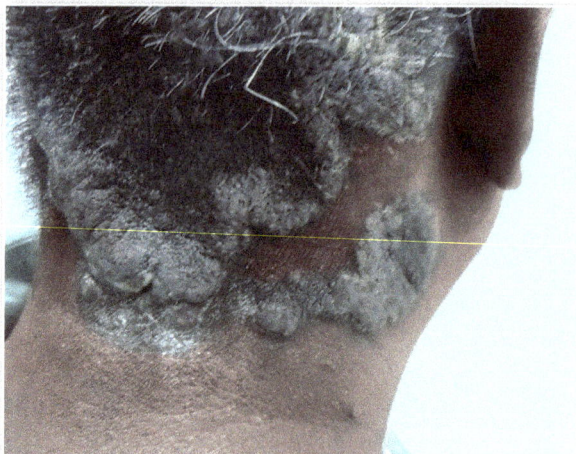

FIG. 73: Tinea corporis extending to the hairy scalp - difficult to diagnose.

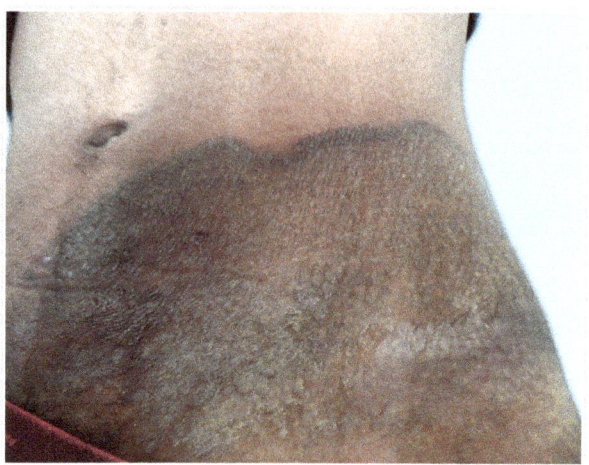

FIG. 74: Noninflammatory tinea corporis over the loin area.

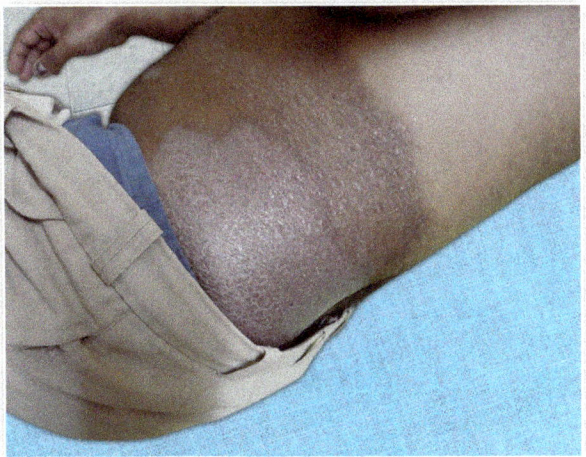

FIG. 75: Psoriasis patient with tinea corporis.

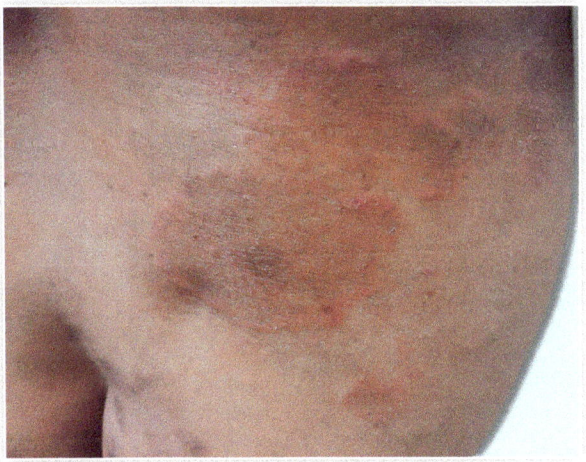

FIG. 76: Recurrence over a partially resolved patch.

Color Atlas of Dermatophytoses: *Focus on Superficial Fungal Infections*

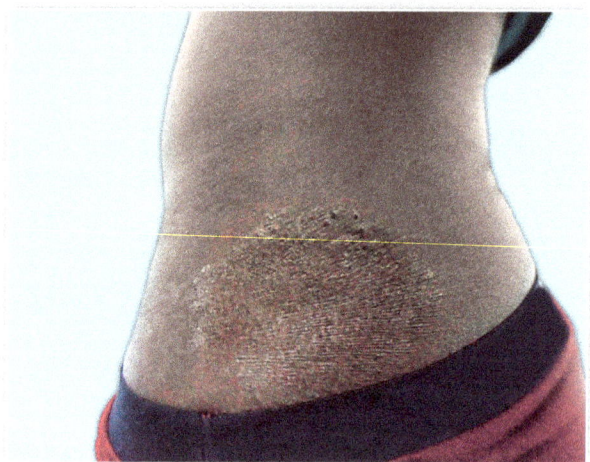

FIG. 77: Scaly patch without central clearance.

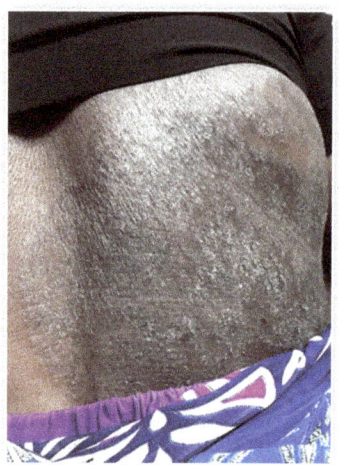

FIG. 78: Large well-defined patch of tinea corporis over the back.

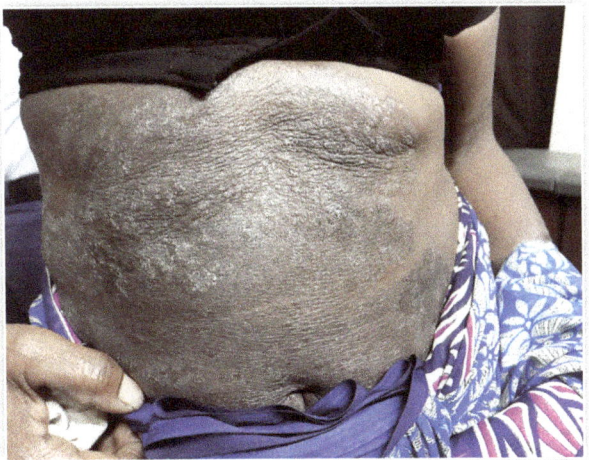

FIG. 79: Same patient as in figure 78.

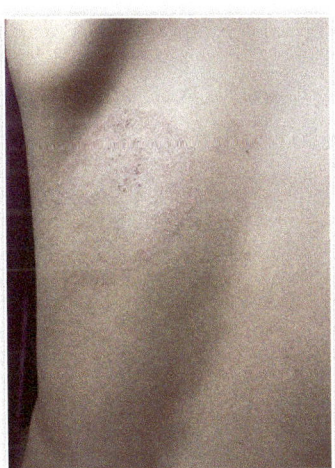

FIG. 80: Ill-defined partially treated patch of tinea corporis.

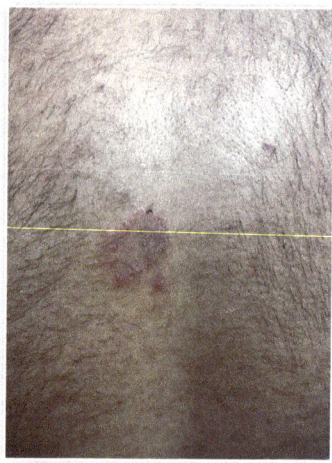

FIG. 81: Classical annular patch with peripheral scaling.

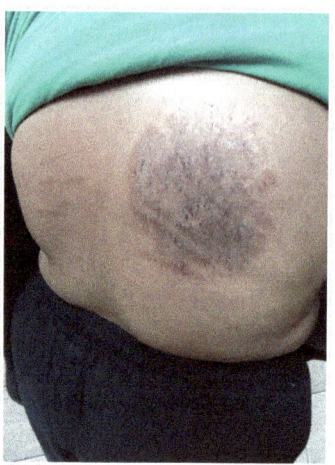

FIG. 82: Irregular margin in a patient treated with steroid combination.

Trunk and Limbs Infection

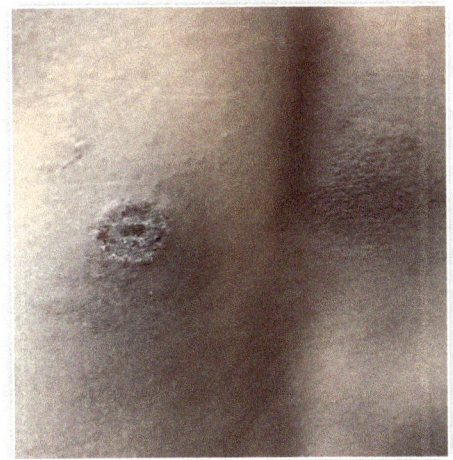

FIG. 83: Appearance of a fresh patch over the resolving area.

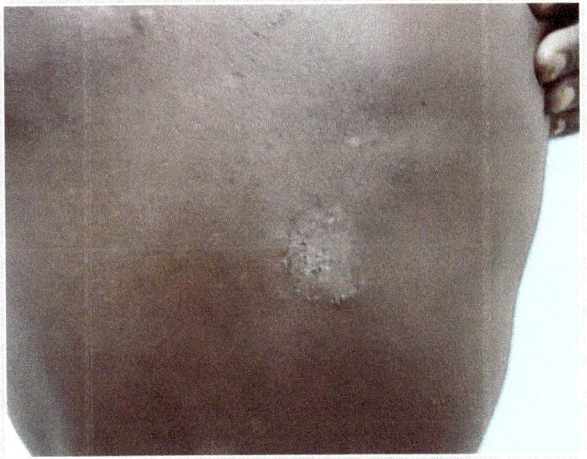

FIG. 84: Partially treated tinea corporis posing diagnostic difficulty.

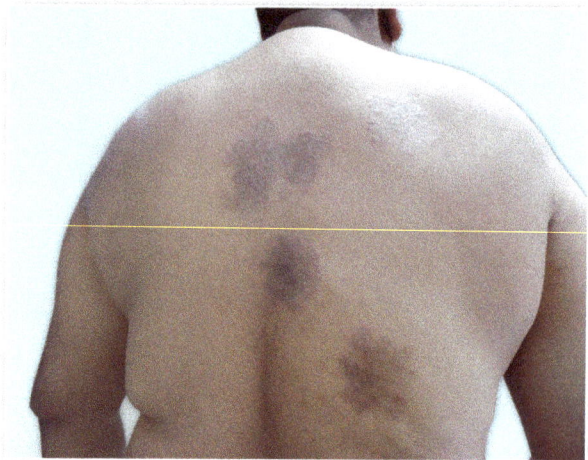

FIG. 85: Multiple patches of tinea corporis over back.

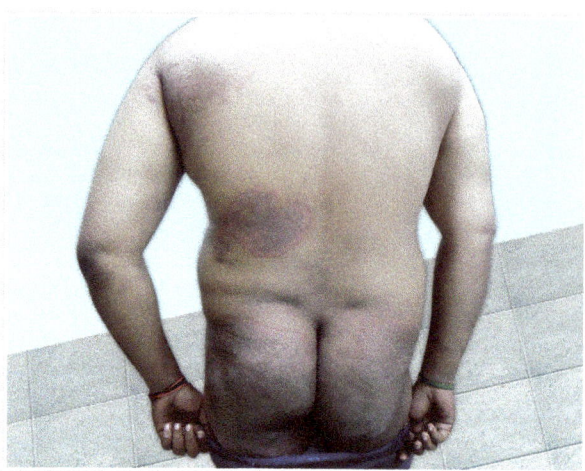

FIG. 86: Tinea corporis with involvement of gluteal region.

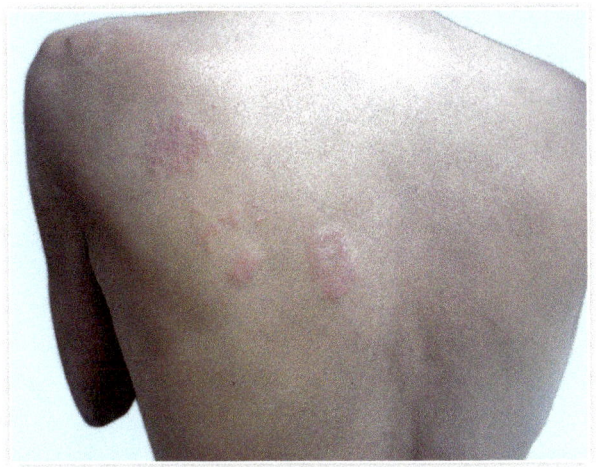

FIG. 87: Multiple patches of tinea corporis.

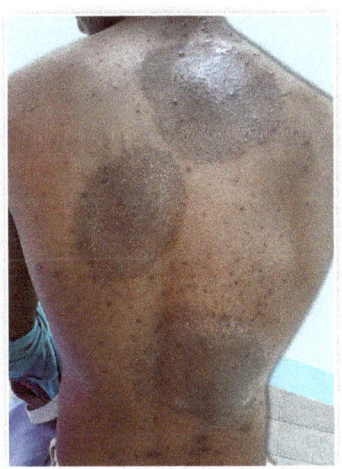

FIG. 88: Extensive involvement of the back in a diabetic patient.

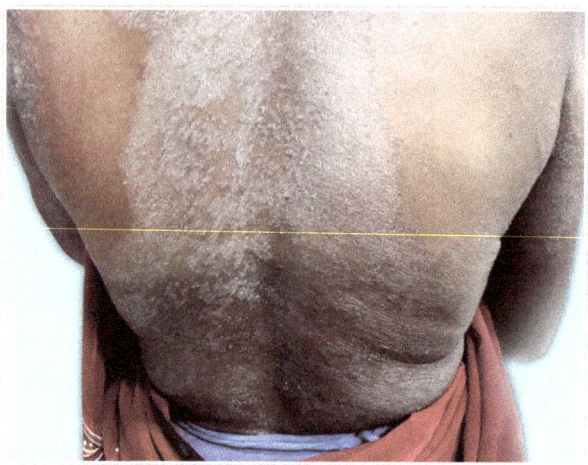

FIG. 89: Same patient as in figure 88.

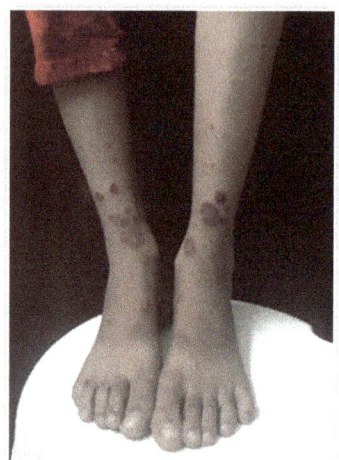

FIG. 90: Tinea corporis involving both legs.

Trunk and Limbs Infection

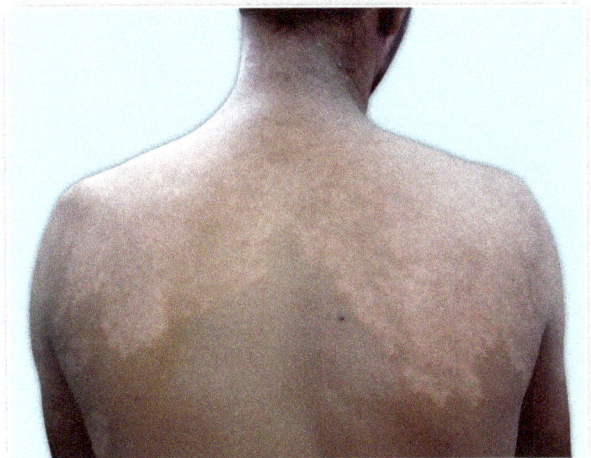

FIG. 91: Upper back involvement in a patient with pityriasis versicolor.

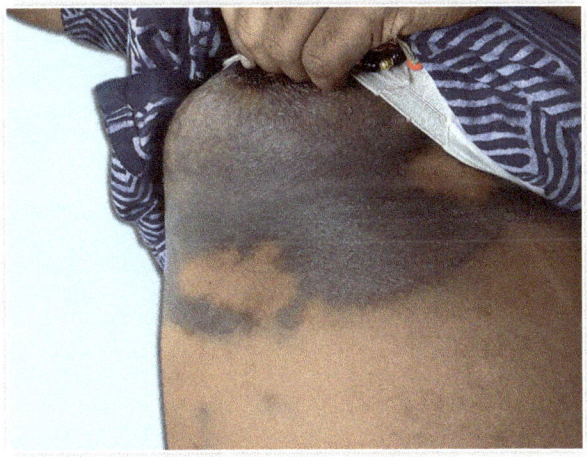

FIG. 92: The classical erythematous advancing margin.

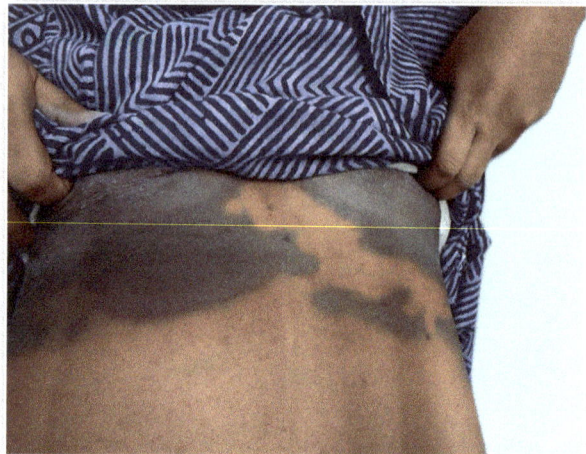

FIG. 93: Involvement of inframammary area.

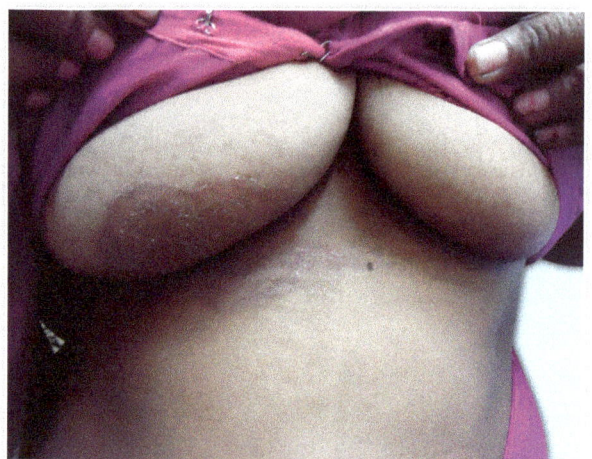

FIG. 94: The unilateral affection.

Trunk and Limbs Infection

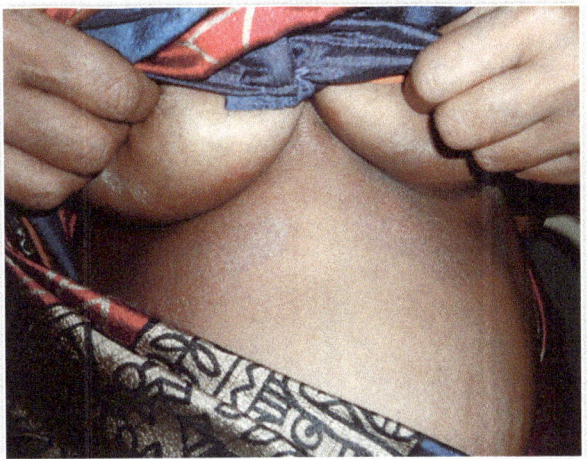

FIG. 95: Bilateral involvement mimicking erythrasma.

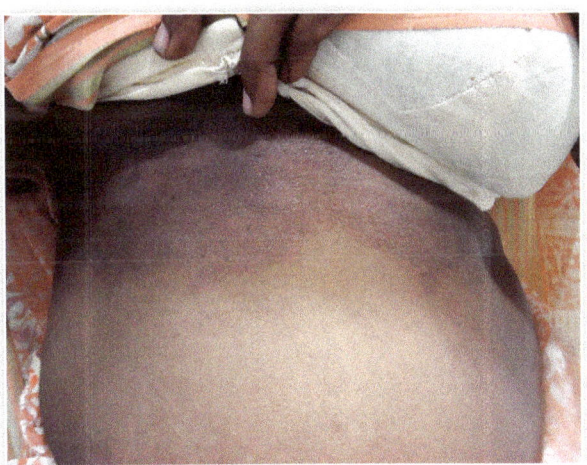

FIG. 96: Inframammary involvement before treatment.

Color Atlas of Dermatophytoses: *Focus on Superficial Fungal Infections*

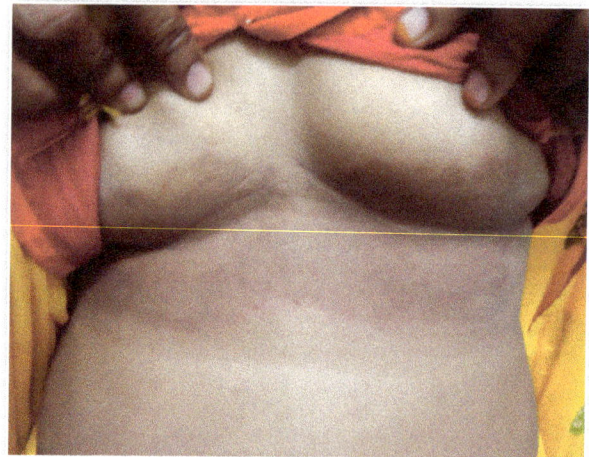

FIG. 97: Same patient as in figure 96 after treatment.

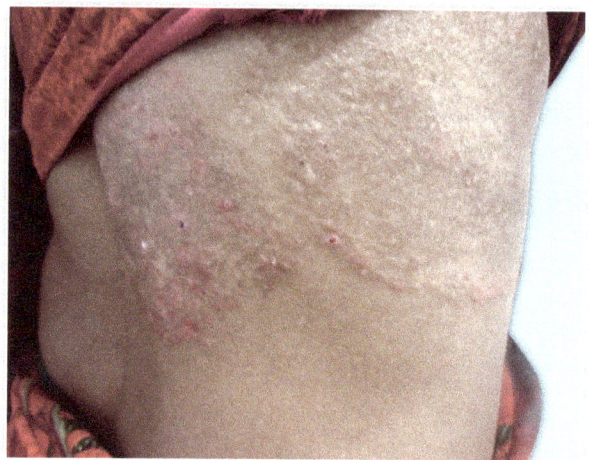

FIG. 98: Extension of inframammary involvement on to the back.

Trunk and Limbs Infection

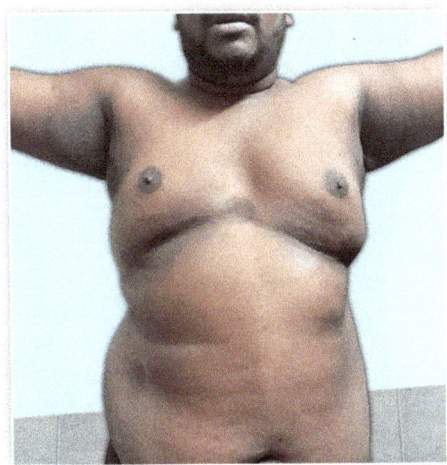

FIG. 99: Inframammary and axillary involvement in an obese male.

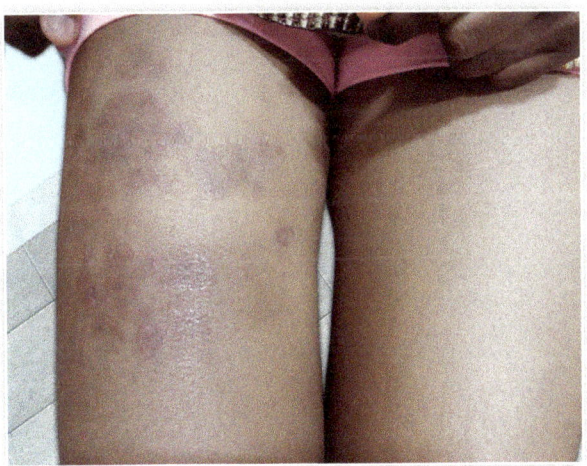

FIG. 100: Tinea corporis of the thigh, note the unilateral involvement.

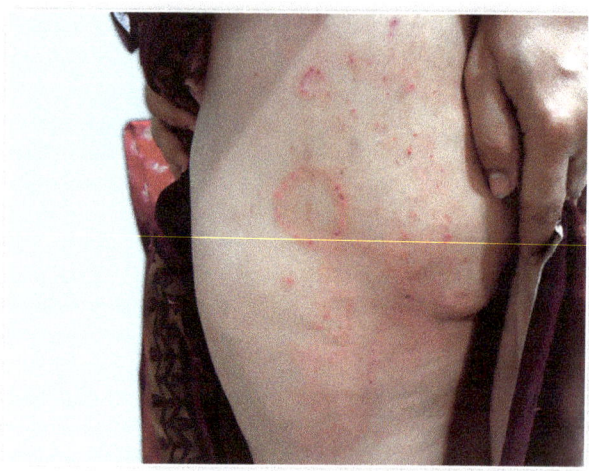

FIG. 101: Tinea incognito where the original morphology is almost lost.

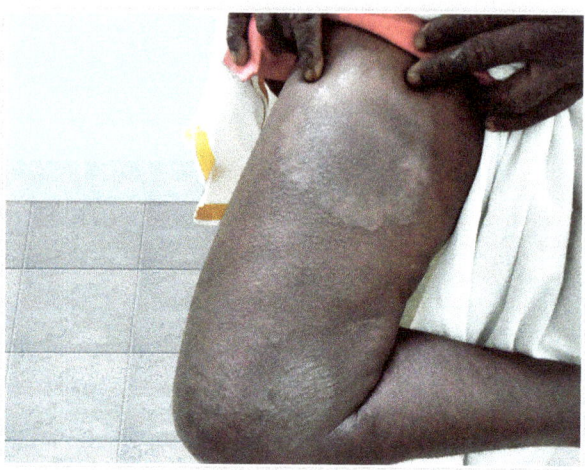

FIG. 102: Classical tinea with central clearing.

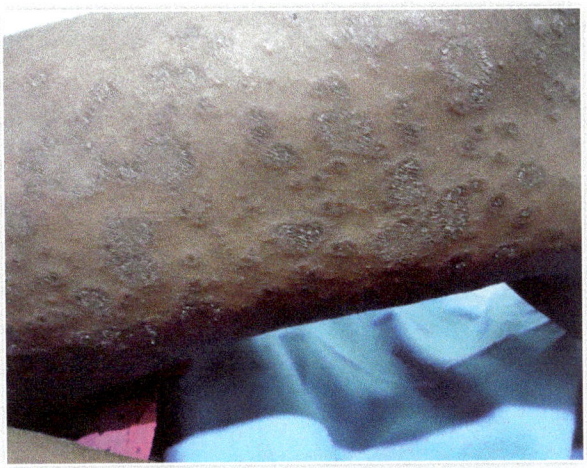

FIG. 103: Multiple small patches mimicking pityriasis rosea.

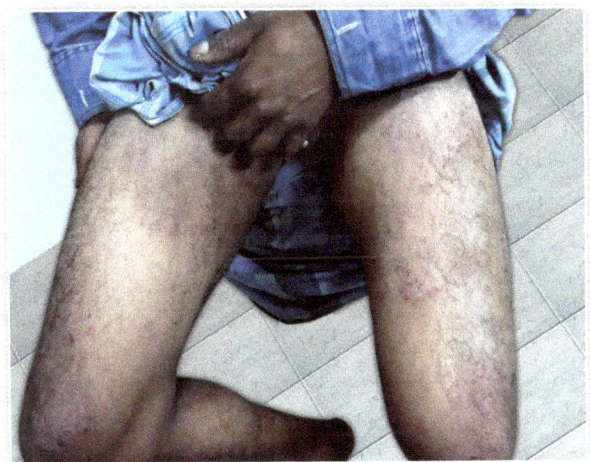

FIG. 104: Bilateral extensive involvement in an immunocompromised.

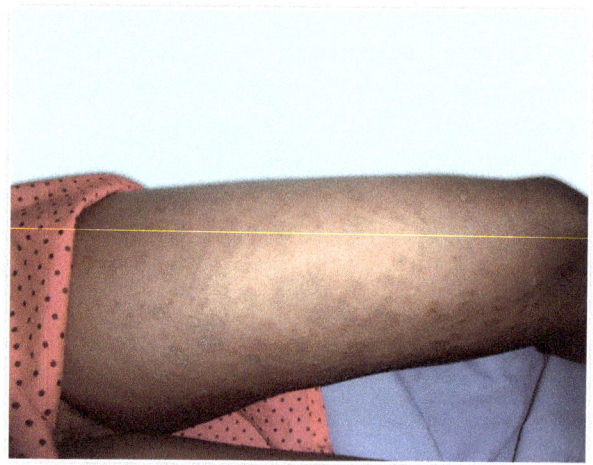

FIG. 105: Treated as pityriasis rosea with topical steroid.

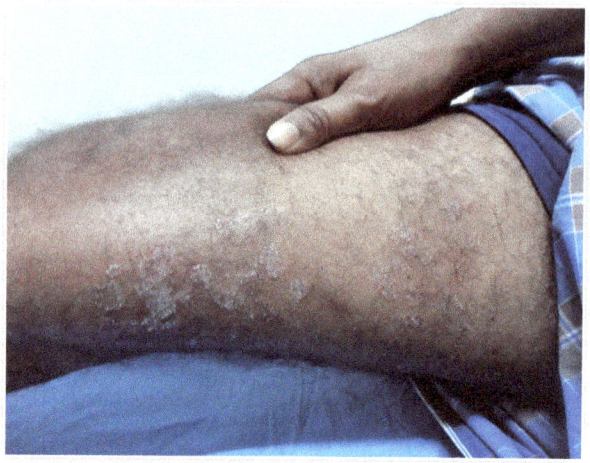

FIG. 106: Multiple small scaly patches.

Trunk and Limbs Infection

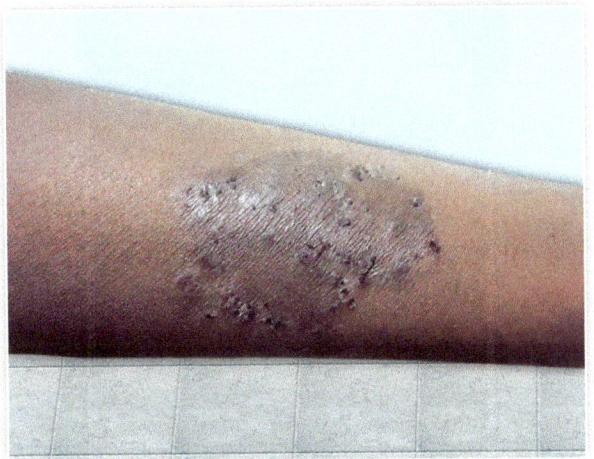

FIG. 107: Crusting over patch of tinea corporis.

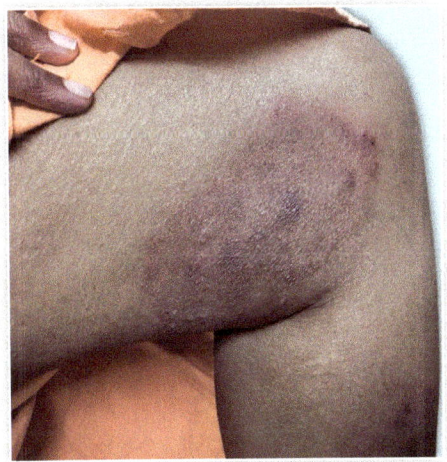

FIG. 108: Activity indicating the need to continue treatment.

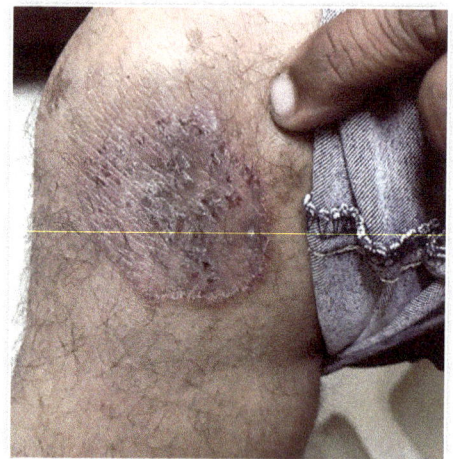

FIG. 109: Erosion over patch.

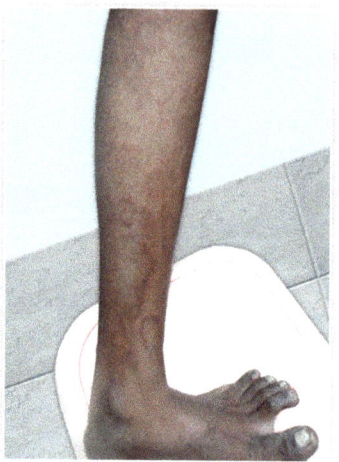

FIG. 110: Multiple small patches over the leg.

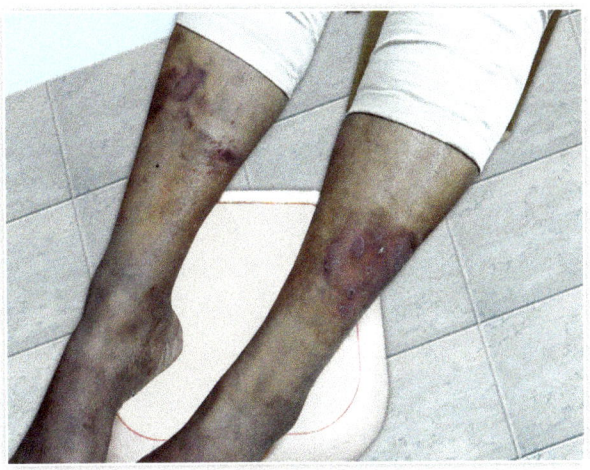

FIG. 111: Erythema secondary to whitfield application.

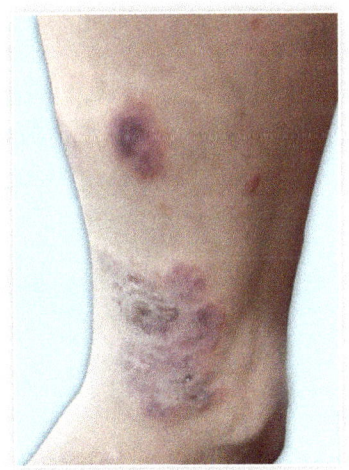

FIG. 112: Multiple small patches.

Color Atlas of Dermatophytoses: *Focus on Superficial Fungal Infections*

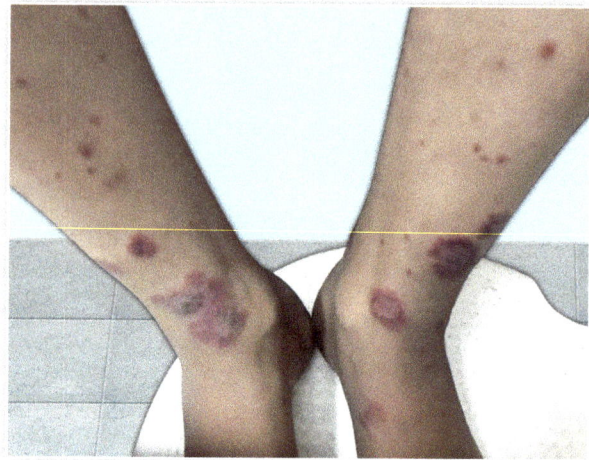

FIG. 113: Same patient as in figure 112.

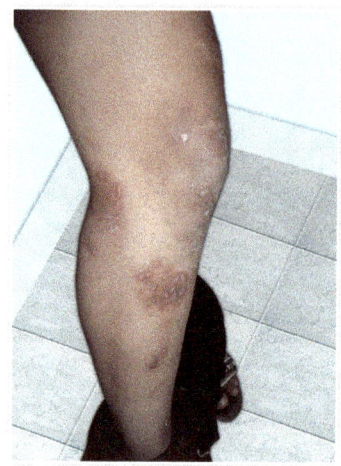

FIG. 114: Multiple crusts over the patch of tinea corporis of the leg.

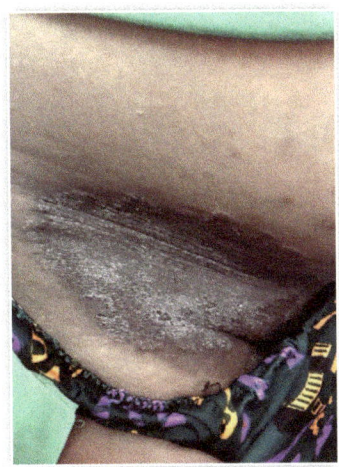

FIG. 115: The pigmentation, scaling and well-defined margin.

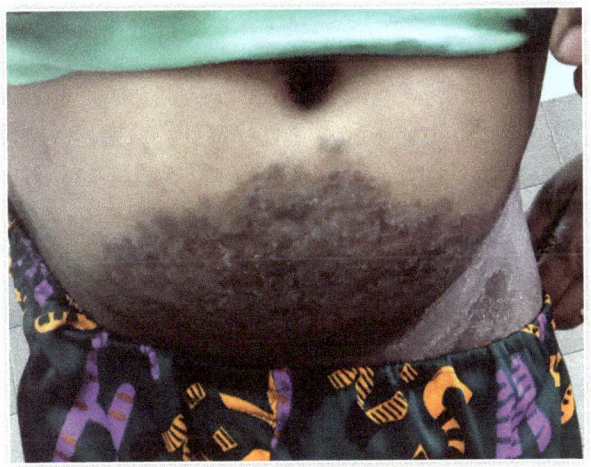

FIG. 116: Same patient as in figure 115.

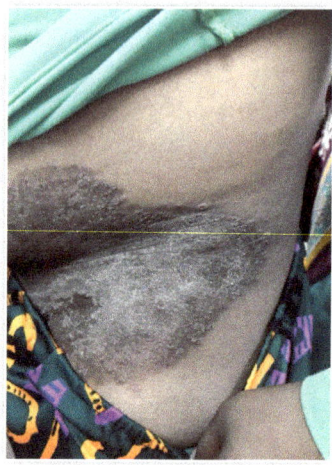

FIG. 117: Same patient as in figure 115.

CHAPTER 4: Axillary Infections

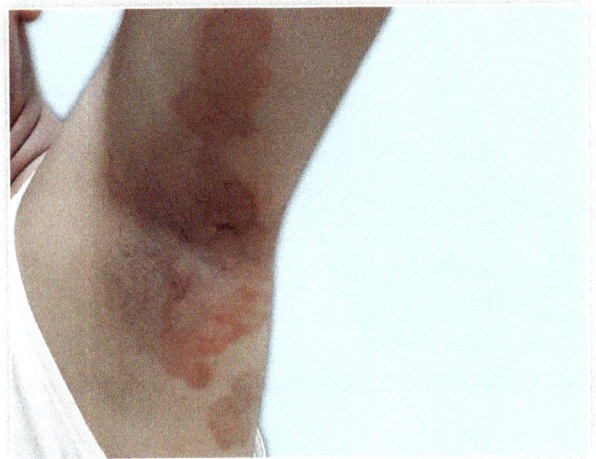

FIG. 1: Tinea axillaris mimicking erythrasma.

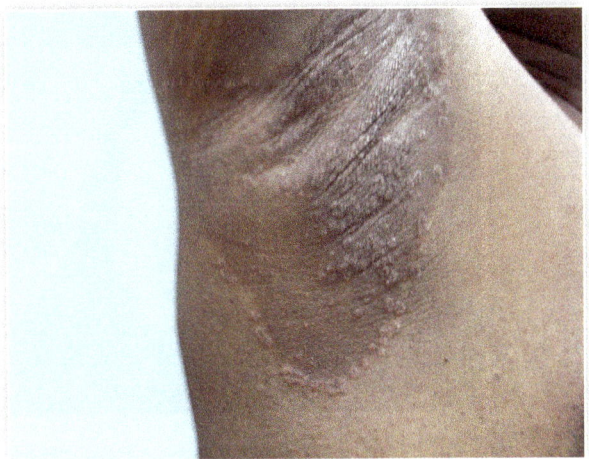

FIG. 2: Tinea axillaris in a patient with acanthosis nigricans.

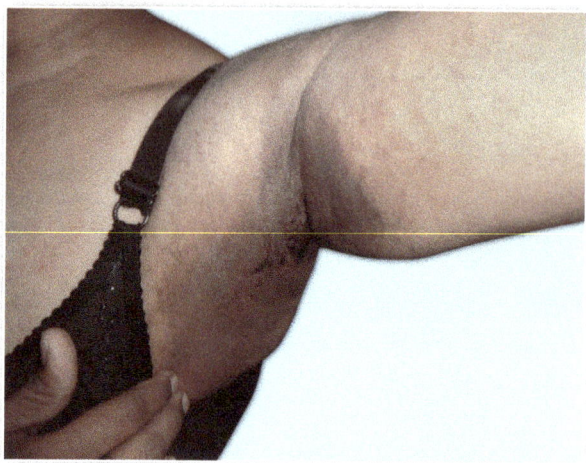

FIG. 3: Tinea axillaris in a diabetic patient mimicking erythrasma.

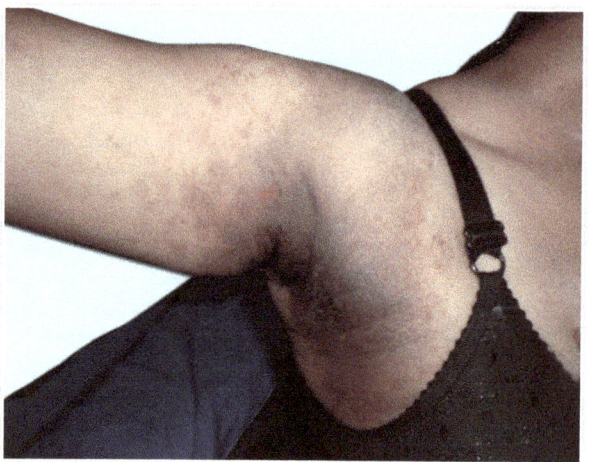

FIG. 4: Same patient as in figure 3.

Axillary Infections

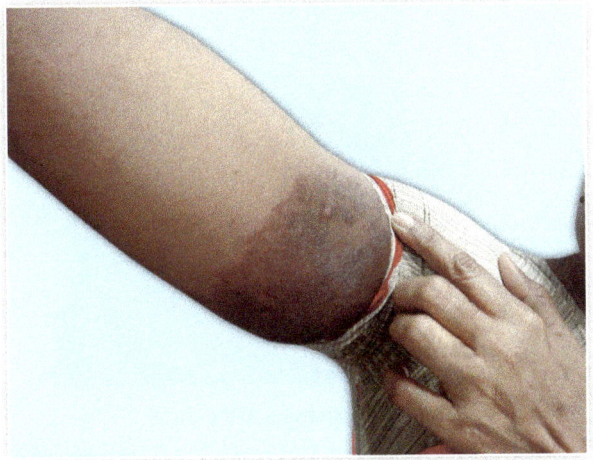

FIG. 5: Tinea axillaris extending on to the arm.

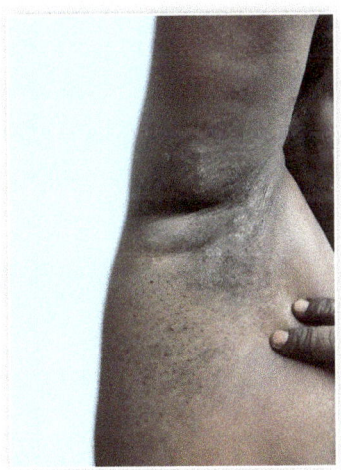

FIG. 6: Multiple small patches in the axilla.

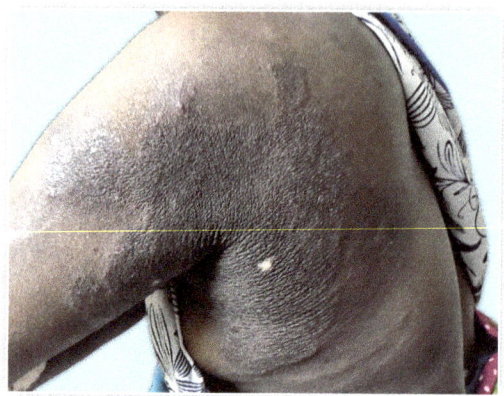

FIG. 7: Tinea axillaris with extension to the chest.

CHAPTER 5

Hand Infections

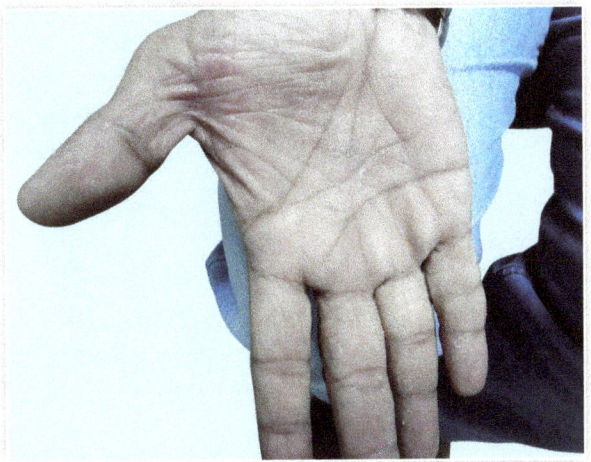

FIG. 1: Tinea manuum involving right hand.

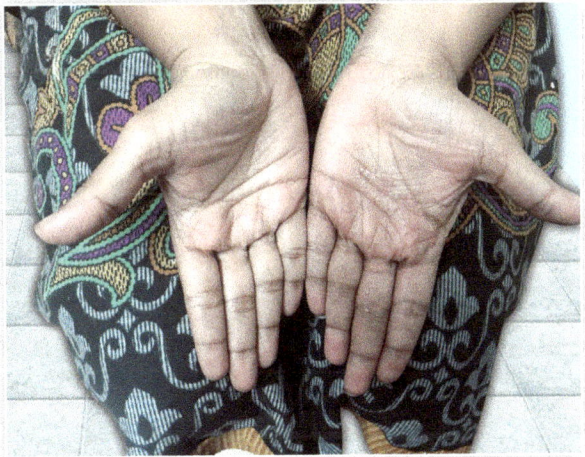

FIG. 2: Same patient as in figure 1. Note scaling over the left palm.

Color Atlas of Dermatophytoses: *Focus on Superficial Fungal Infections*

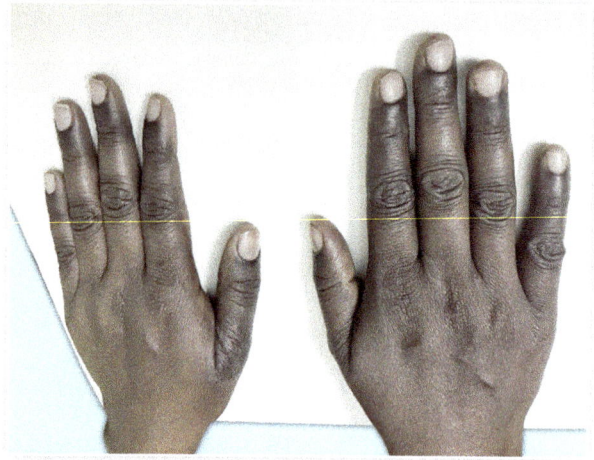

FIG. 3: Tinea manuum involving the left thumb.

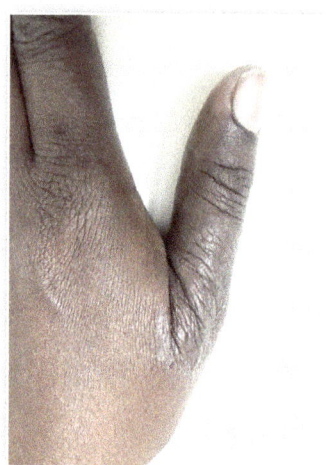

FIG. 4: Same patient as figure 3. Note the well-defined margin.

Hand Infections

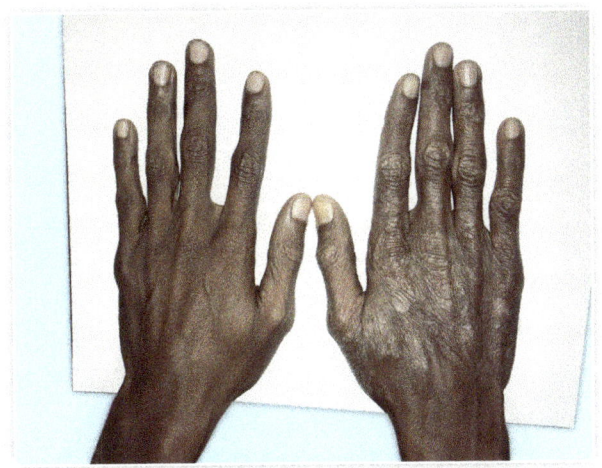

FIG. 5: Tinea manuum of the right dorsum.

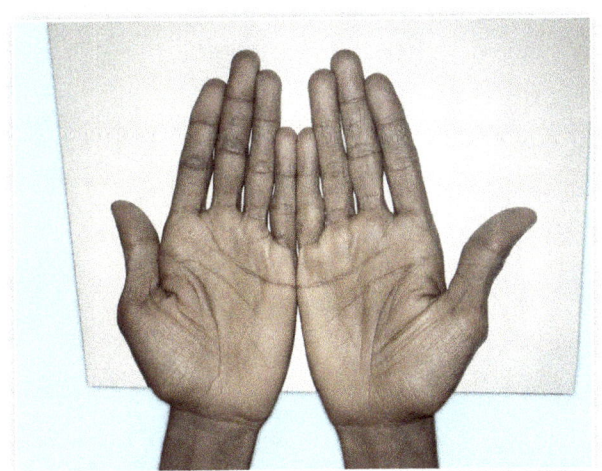

FIG. 6: Same patient as in figure 5. Note sparing of the palmar surface.

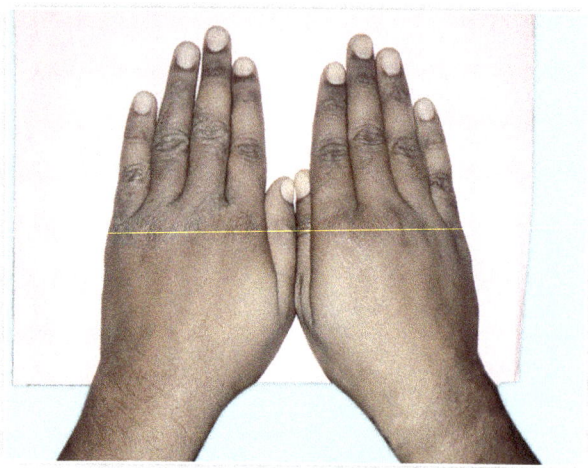

FIG. 7: Tinea manuum of the left hand dorsal aspect.

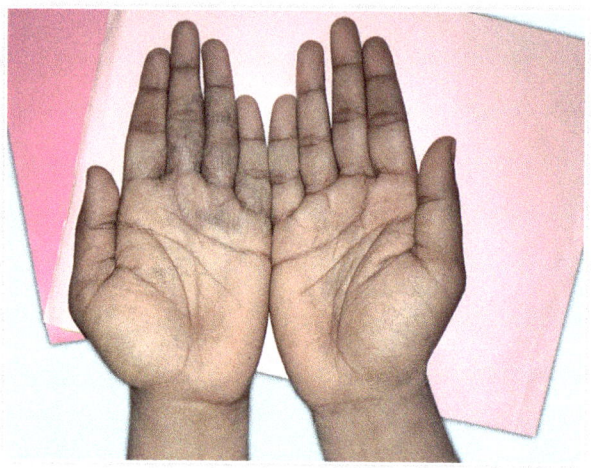

FIG. 8: Same patient as in figure 7 showing involvement of the palmar skin.

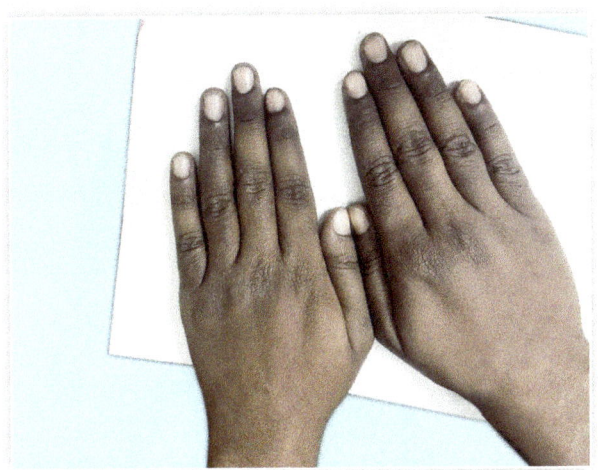

FIG. 9: Same patient as in figure 7 after treatment.

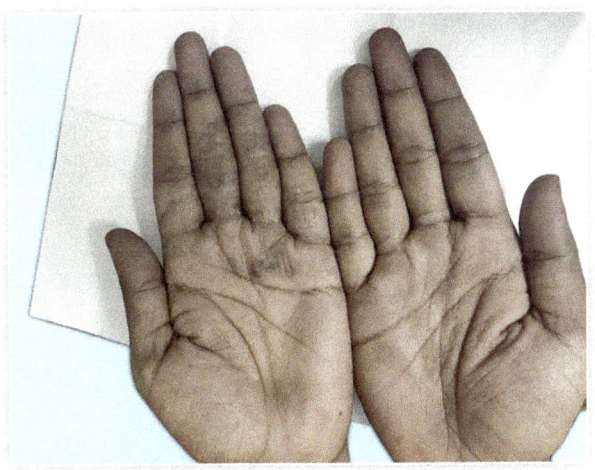

FIG. 10: Same patient as in figure 8 after treatment.

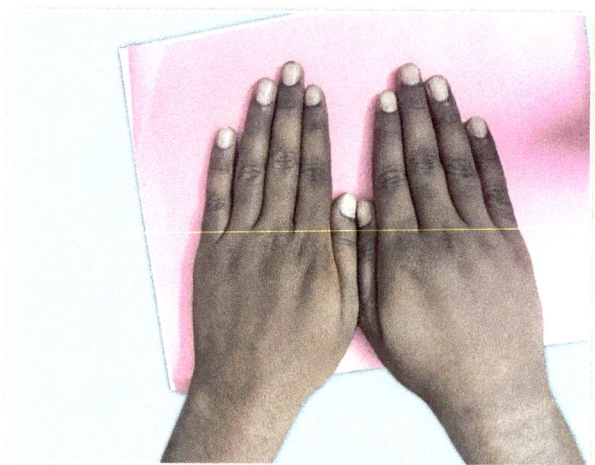

FIG. 11: Same patient as in figure 9 after complete treatment.

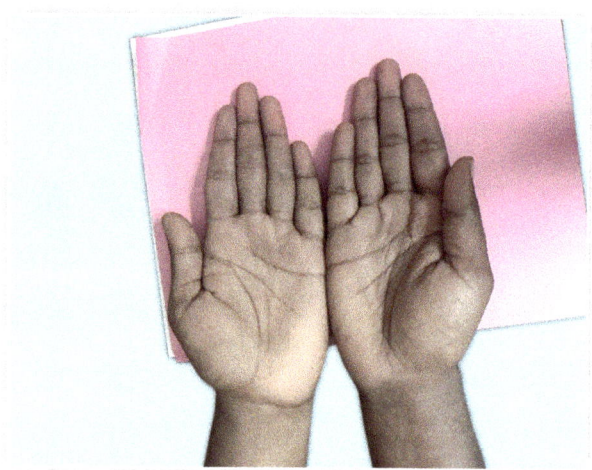

FIG. 12: Same patient as in figure 10 scraping negative after treatment.

Hand Infections

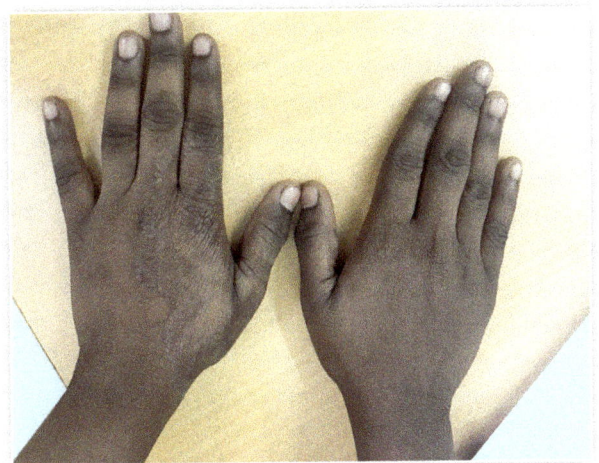

FIG. 13: Tinea manuum in an adolescent which was asymptomatic.

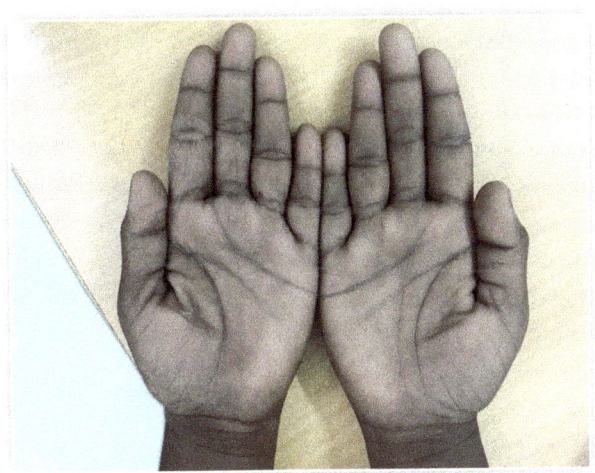

FIG. 14: Same patient as in figure 13.

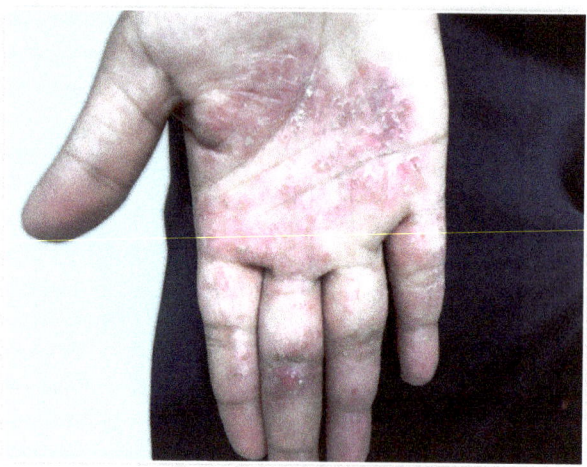

FIG. 15: Retained dermatoglyphics in tinea manuum.

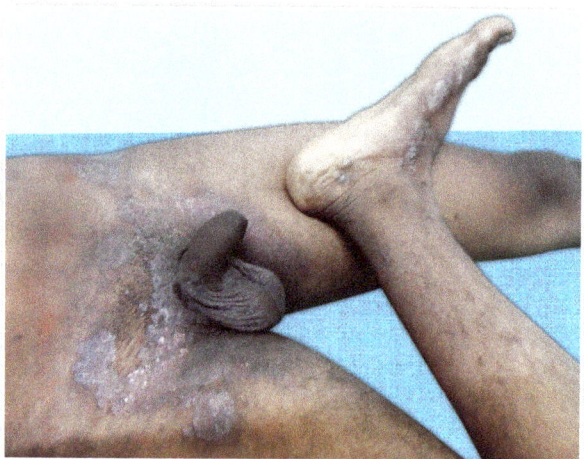

FIG. 16: Tinea pedis with tinea cruris.

Hand Infections

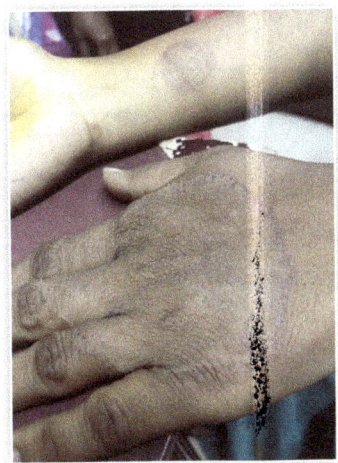

FIG. 17: Tinea manuum in mother and tinea corporis in daughter.

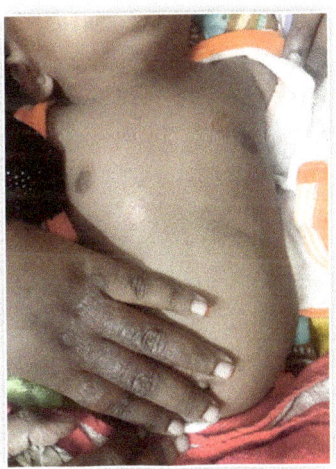

FIG. 18: Tinea manuum in mother with tinea corporis in her child.

CHAPTER 6: Groin Infections

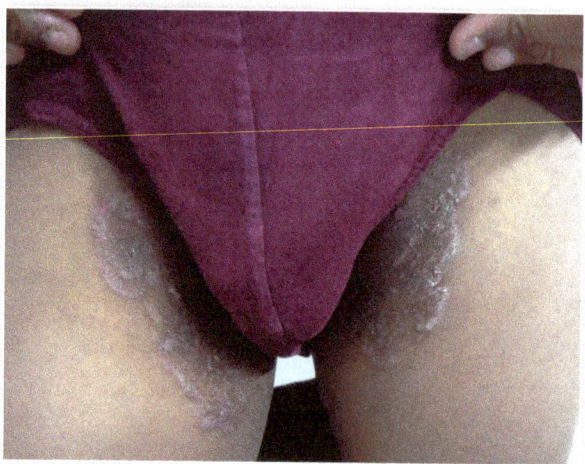

FIG. 1: Classical tinea cruris.

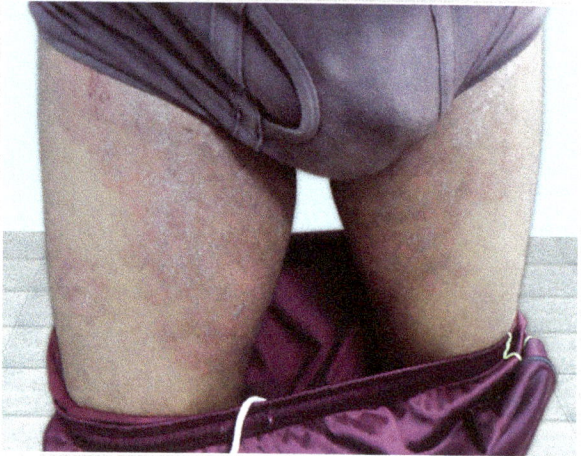

FIG. 2: Tinea cruris extending to almost the entire thigh.

Groin Infections

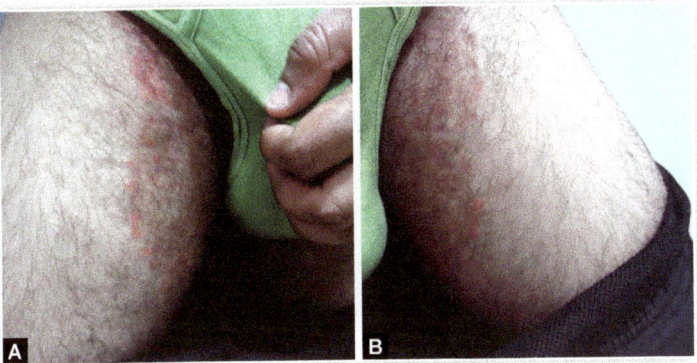

FIGS. 3A AND B: Tinea cruris, note the erythema.

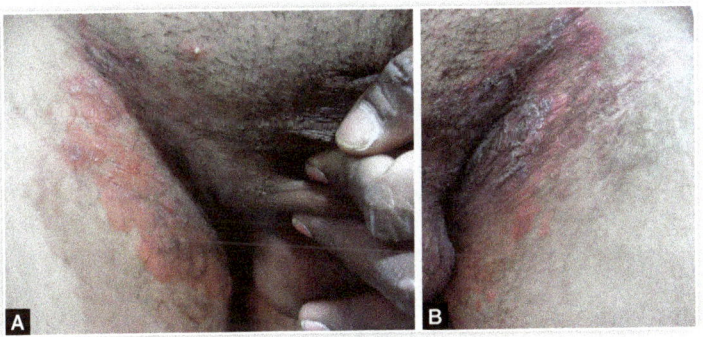

FIGS. 4A AND B: Tinea cruris along with flexural psoriasis.

Color Atlas of Dermatophytoses: *Focus on Superficial Fungal Infections*

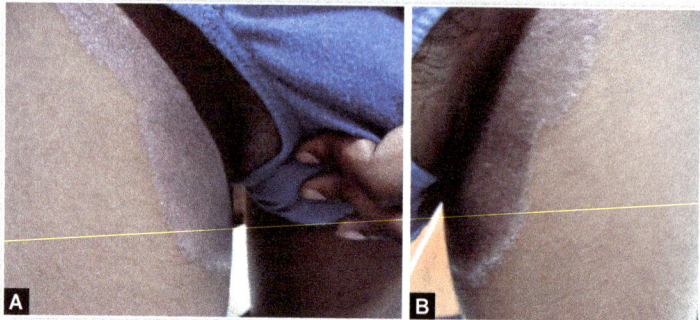

FIGS. 5A AND B: Tinea cruris with active margin.

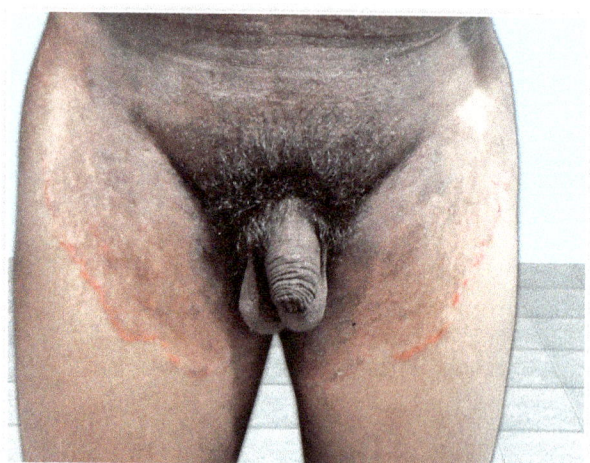

FIG. 6: Recalcitrant tinea cruris and corporis.

Groin Infections

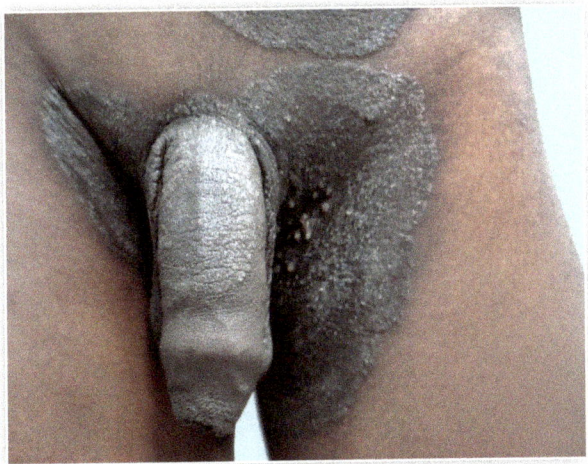

FIG. 7: Tinea cruris with tinea genitalis.

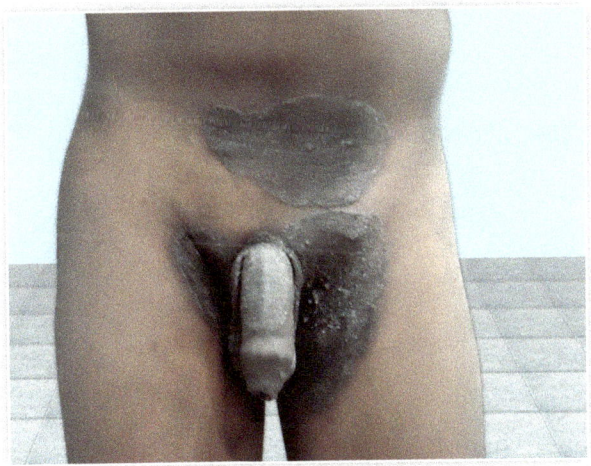

FIG. 8: Same patient as in figure 7 during treatment.

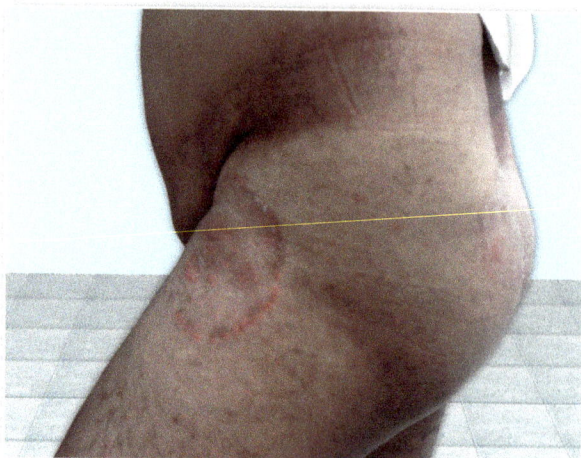

FIG. 9: Patient with tinea cruris showing lesions over the thigh and gluteal area.

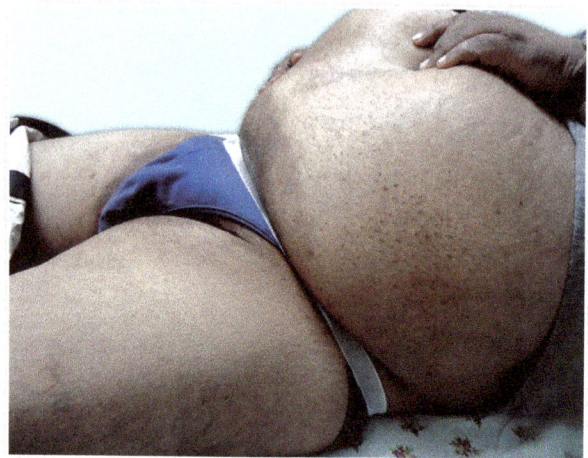

FIG. 10: Tinea cruris and genitalis in an obese man.

Groin Infections

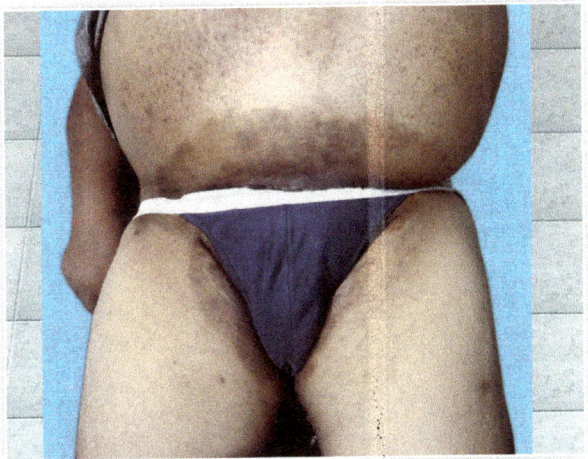

FIG. 11: Same patient as in figure 10 showing extension to the lower abdomen.

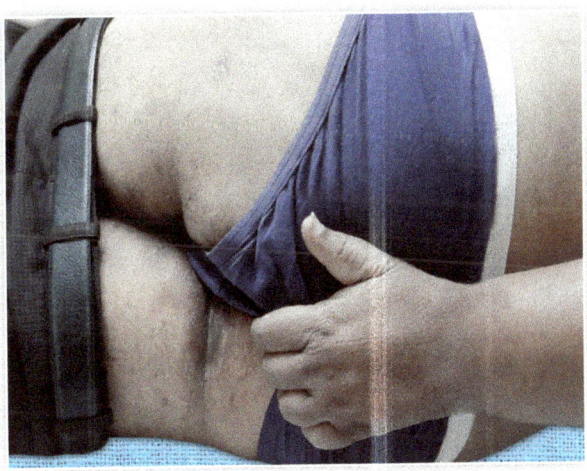

FIG. 12: Same patient as in figures 10 and 11. Note involvement of the folds.

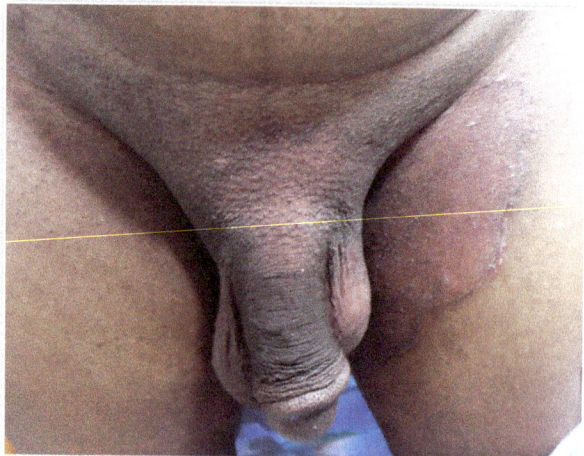

FIG. 13: Unilateral tinea cruris.

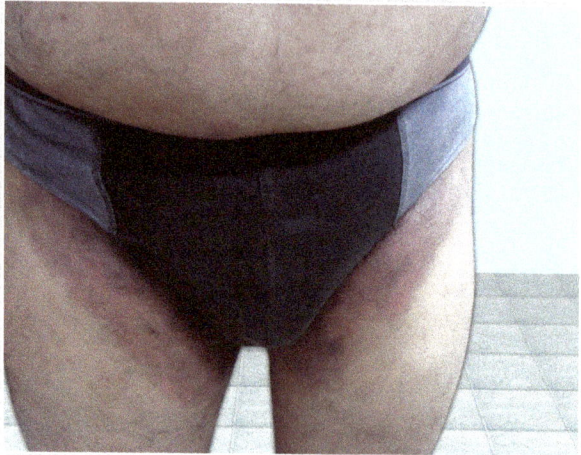

FIG. 14: Post-treatment pigmentation.

Groin Infections

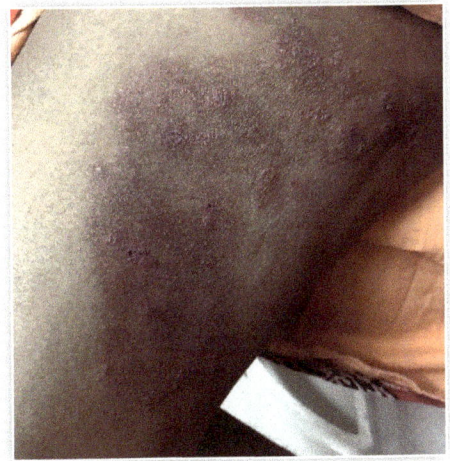

FIG. 15: Involvement of thigh as an extension of tinea cruris.

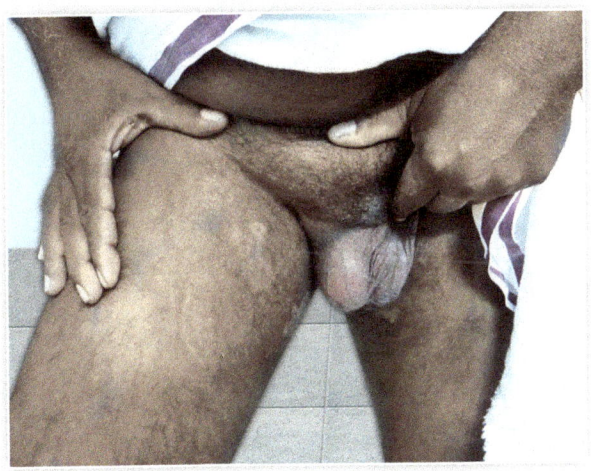

FIG. 16: Tinea cruris with ill-defined margin and involvement of scrotum.

Color Atlas of Dermatophytoses: *Focus on Superficial Fungal Infections*

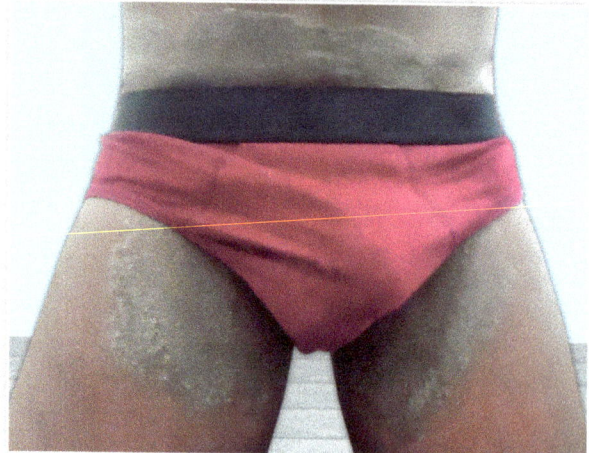

FIG. 17: Extensive involvement of the thigh and lower abdomen.

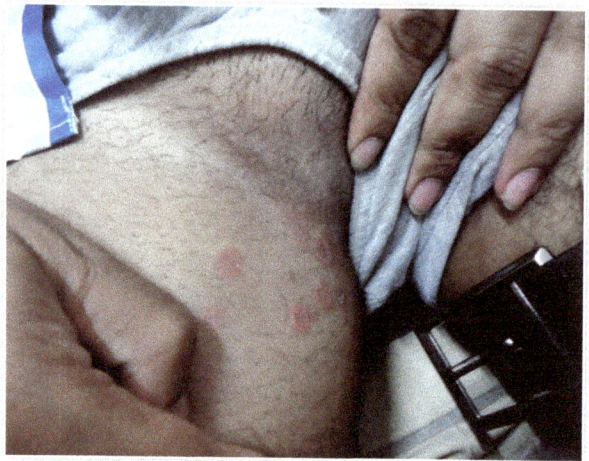

FIG. 18: Multiple small patches of tinea cruris.

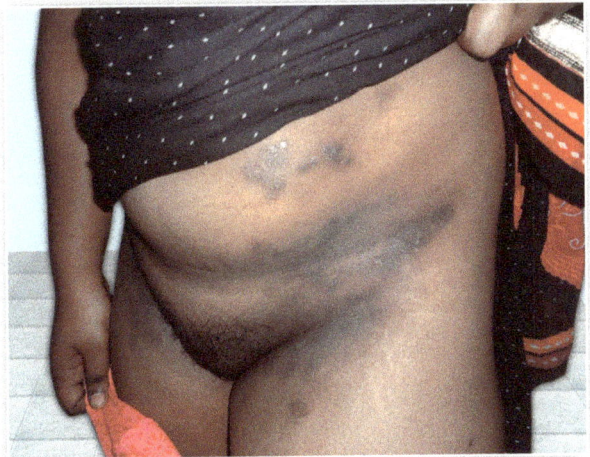

FIG. 19: Tinea cruris with corporis showing hyperpigmenation.

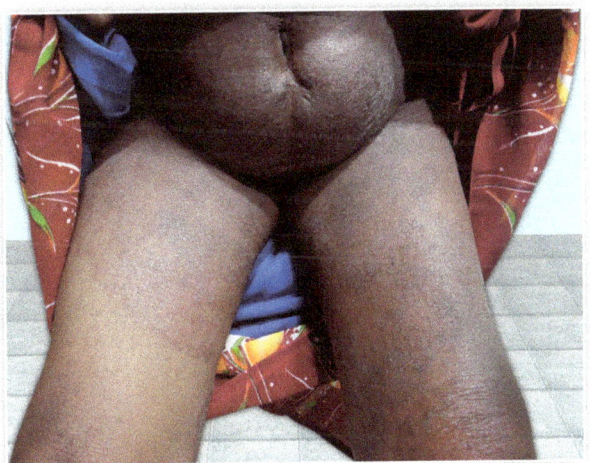

FIG. 20: Extensive dermatophyte infection.

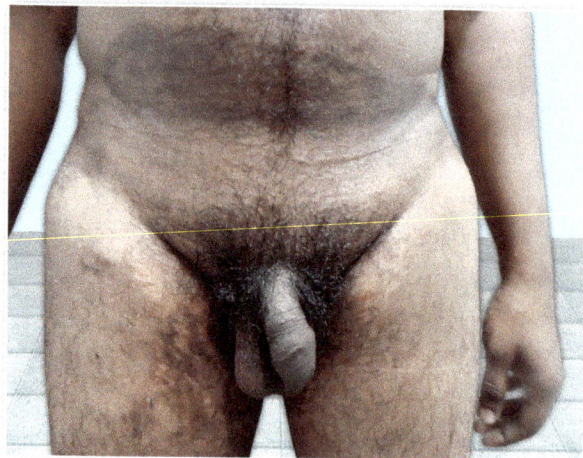

FIG. 21: Genital tinea treated with topical steroids. Note the striae.

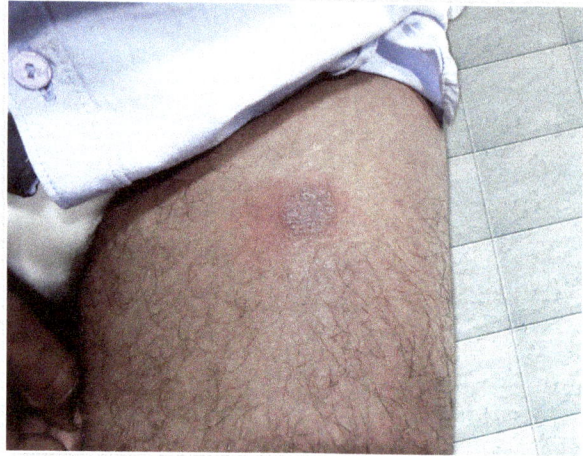

FIG. 22: Single patch over the thigh in a patient treated for tinea cruris.

Groin Infections

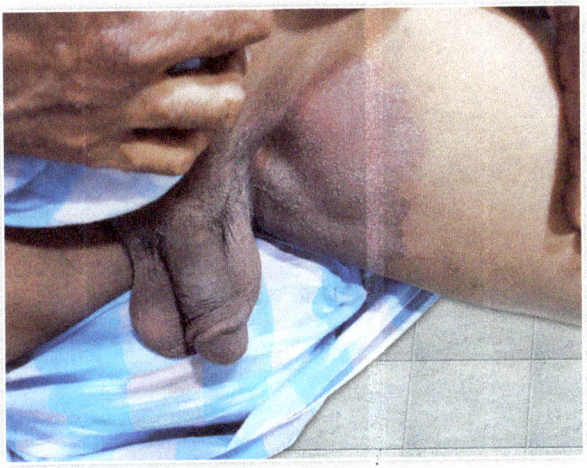

FIG. 23: Tinea cruris mimicking erythrasma.

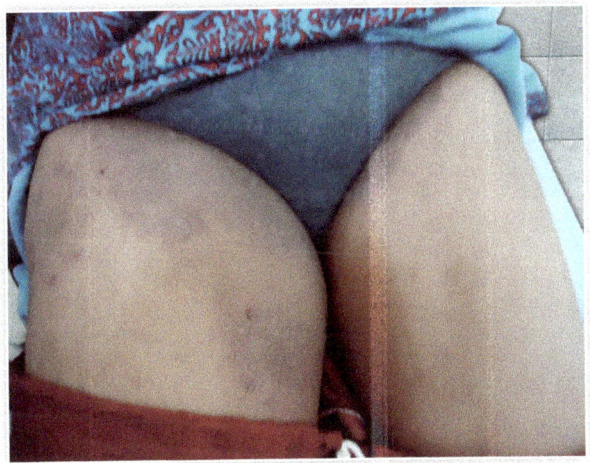

FIG. 24: Postinflammatory pigmentation in a healed patch of tinea cruris.

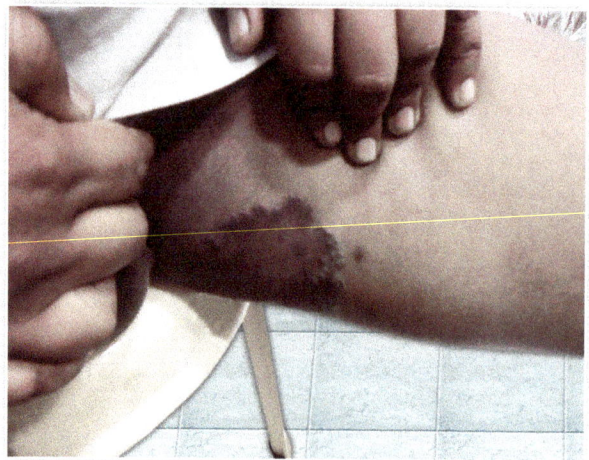

FIG. 25: Tinea cruris with active border.

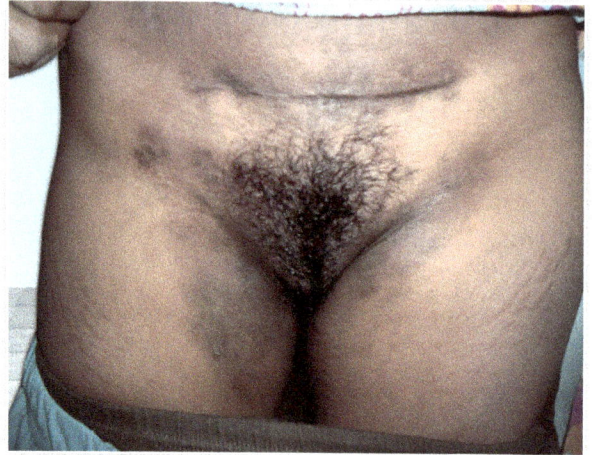

FIG. 26: Tinea cruris in an adolescent.

Groin Infections

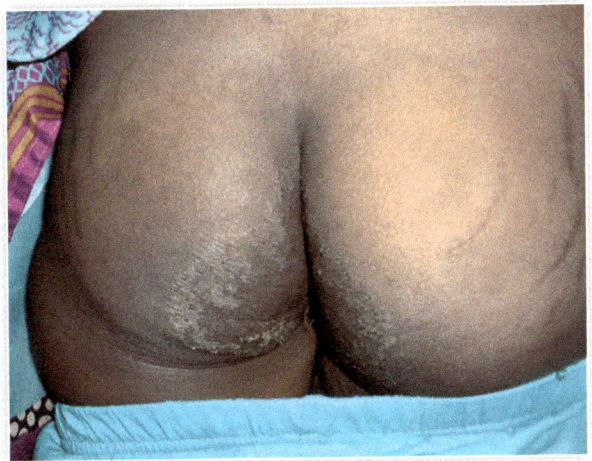

FIG. 27: Same patient as in figure 26.

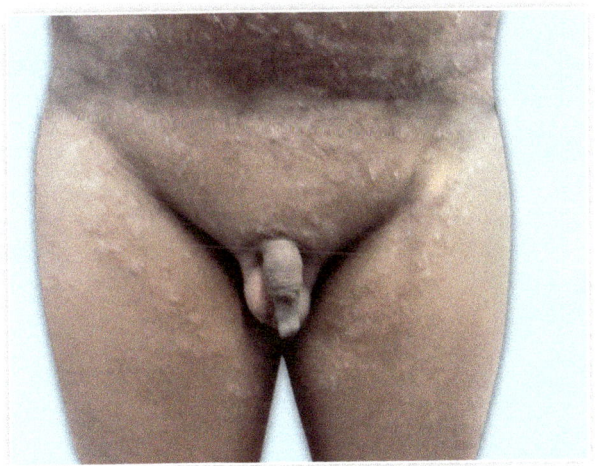

FIG. 28: Tinea cruris, genitalis and corporis in a toddler.

Color Atlas of Dermatophytoses: *Focus on Superficial Fungal Infections*

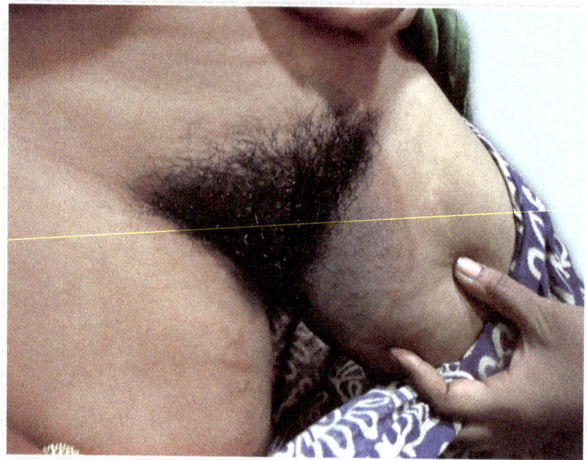

FIG. 29: Involvement of one side alone.

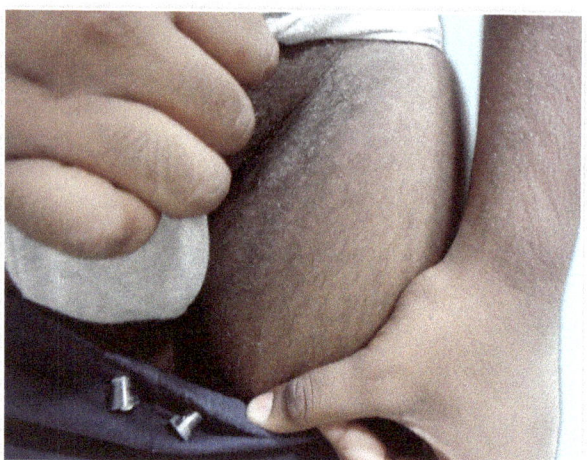

FIG. 30: Very vague patch of tinea cruris, but showing well-defined margin.

Groin Infections

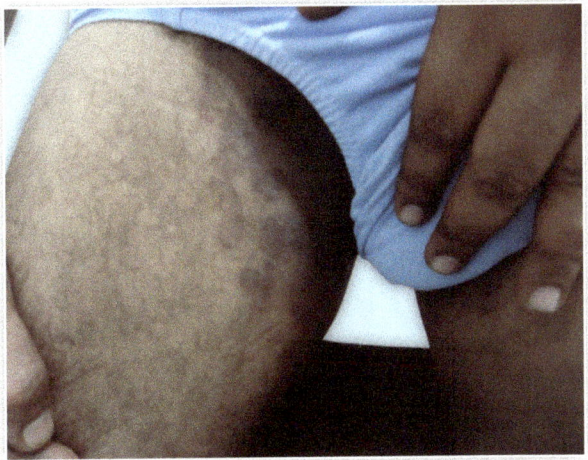

FIG. 31: Tinea cruris in an adult.

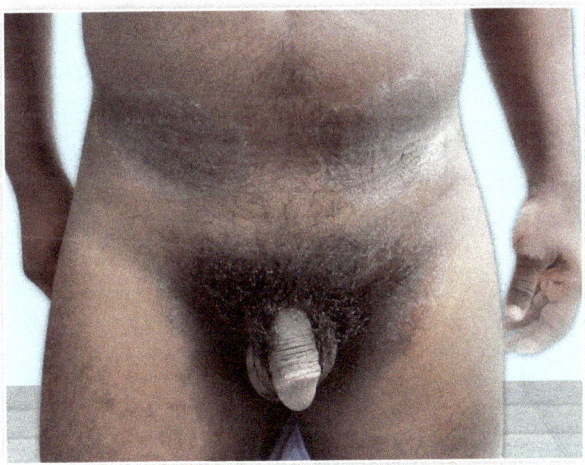

FIG. 32: Tinea cruris with involvement of the waist showing well-defined margin.

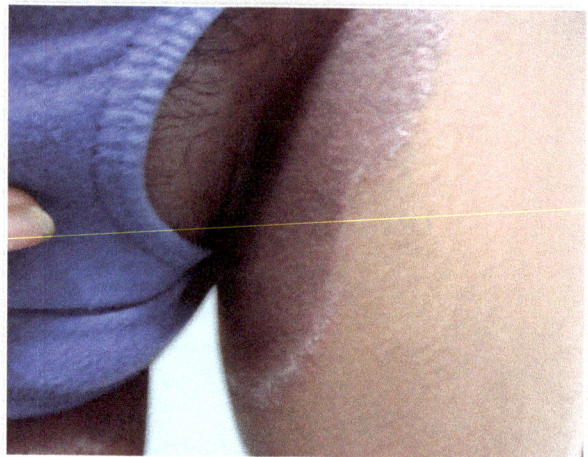

FIG. 33: Classical scaly margin.

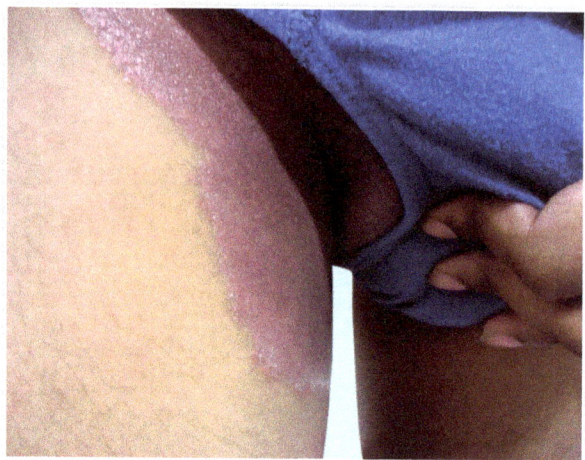

FIG. 34: Same patient as in figure 33.

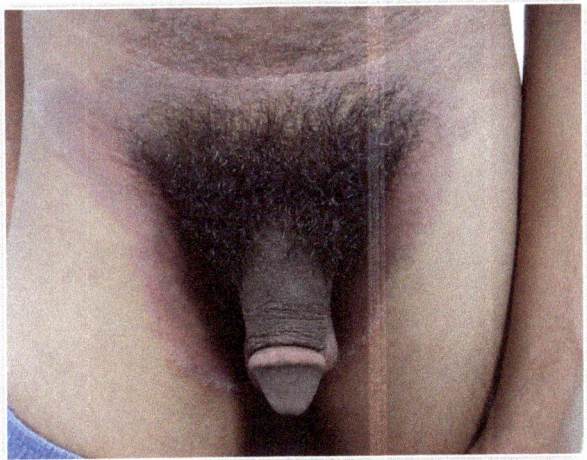

FIG. 35: Same patient as in figures 33 and 34 showing extensive involvement.

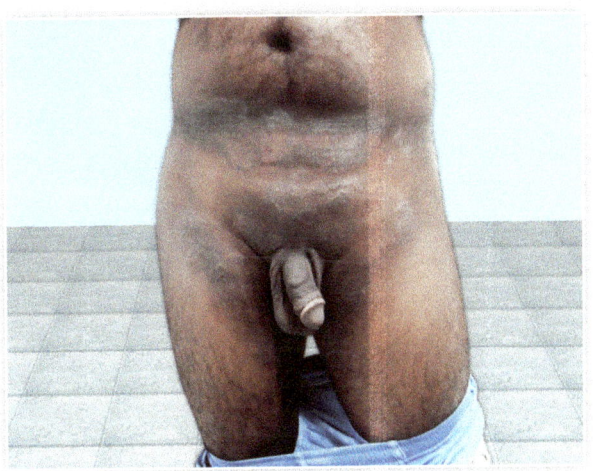

FIG. 36: Widespread dermatophyte infection started as tinea cruris.

Color Atlas of Dermatophytoses: *Focus on Superficial Fungal Infections*

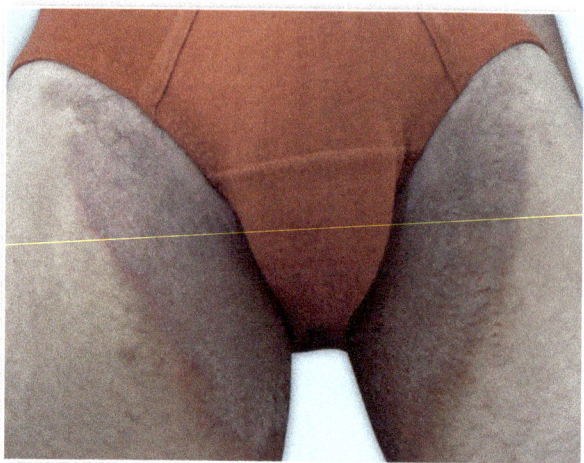

FIG. 37: Tinea cruris with postinflammatory pigmentation and active margin.

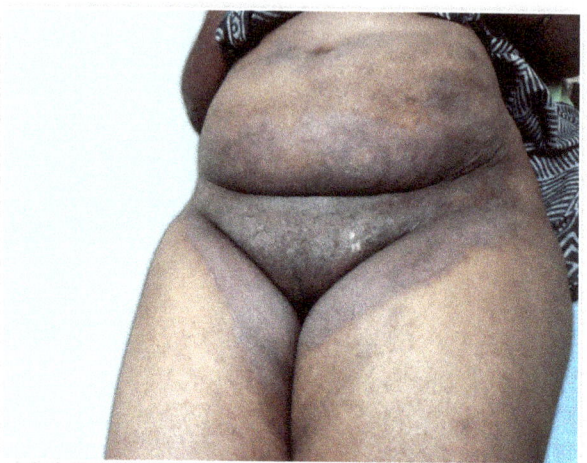

FIG. 38: Tinea cruris in a female.

Groin Infections

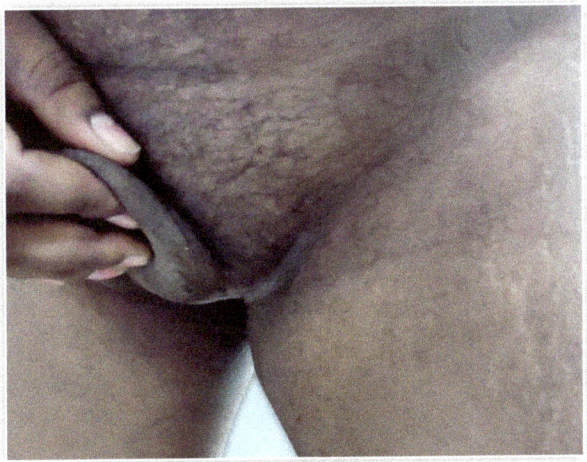

FIG. 39: Patch involving the inguinal fold and part of scrotum.

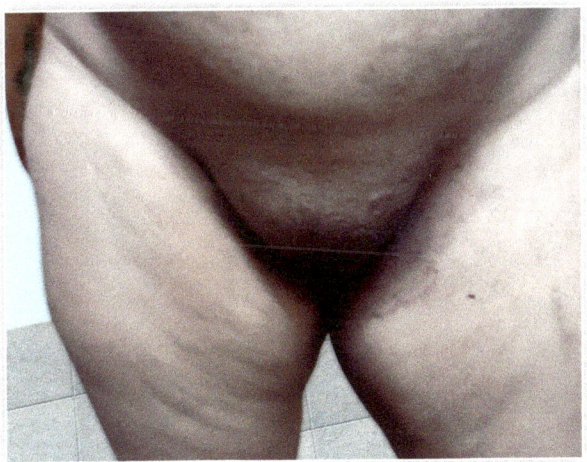

FIG. 40: Tinea cruris also involving the genital area.

Color Atlas of Dermatophytoses: *Focus on Superficial Fungal Infections*

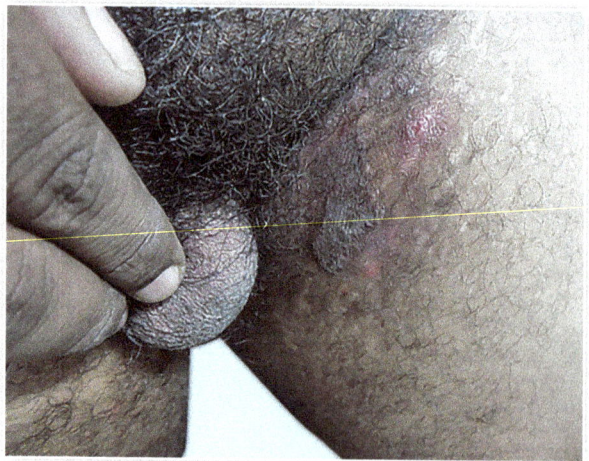

FIG. 41: Intense erythema following an irritant application.

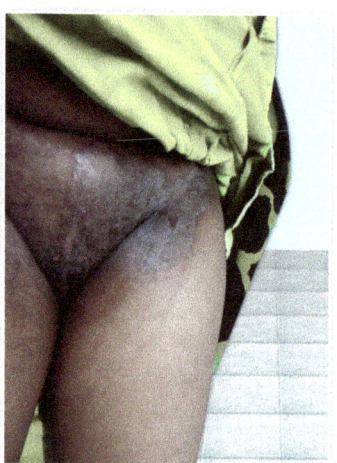

FIG. 42: Classical tinea cruris but almost not crossing midline.

Groin Infections

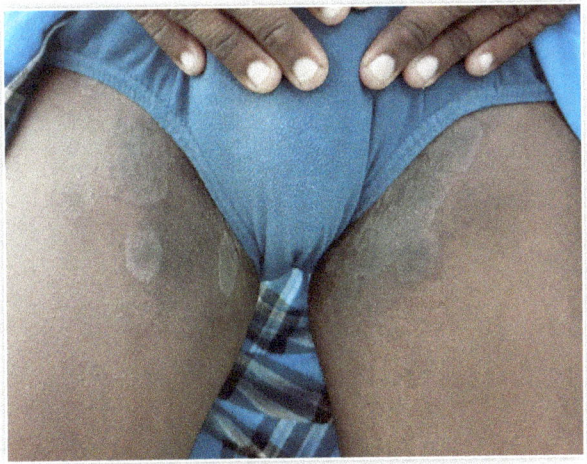

FIG. 43: Tinea cruris in a male.

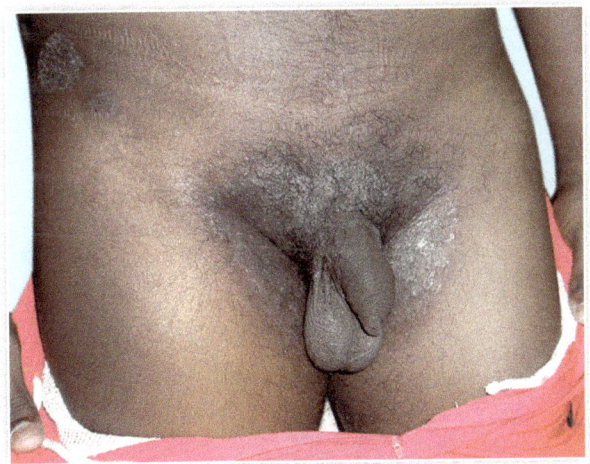

FIG. 44: Tinea cruris in a young boy, note patch over waist.

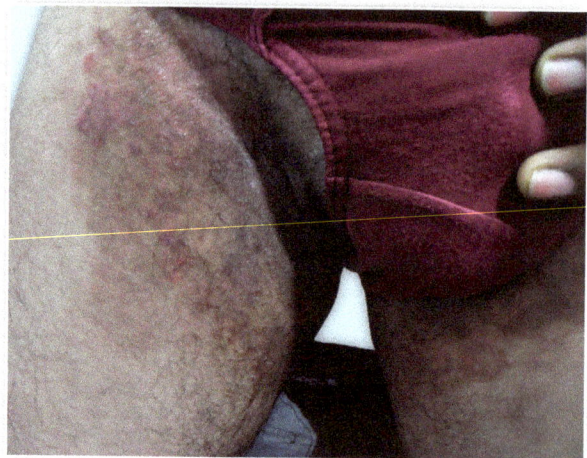

FIG. 45: Tinea cruris showing erythema over new patches.

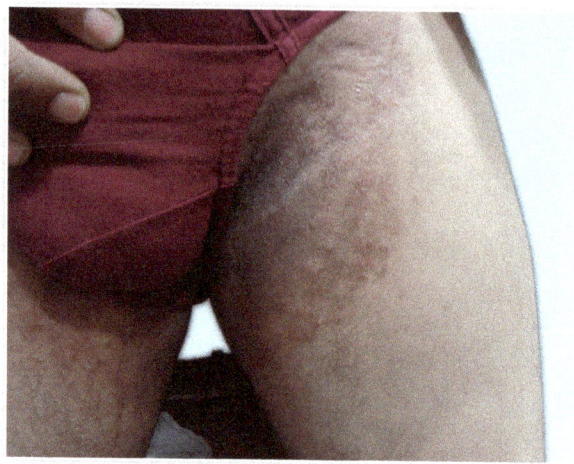

FIG. 46: Same patient as in figure 45.

Groin Infections

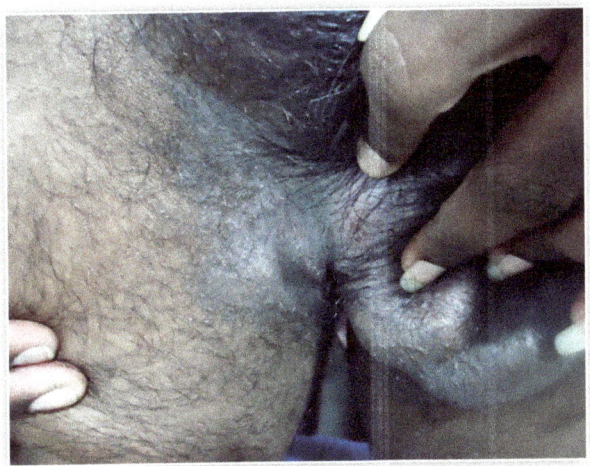

FIG. 47: Tinea cruris showing lichenification not a classical presentation.

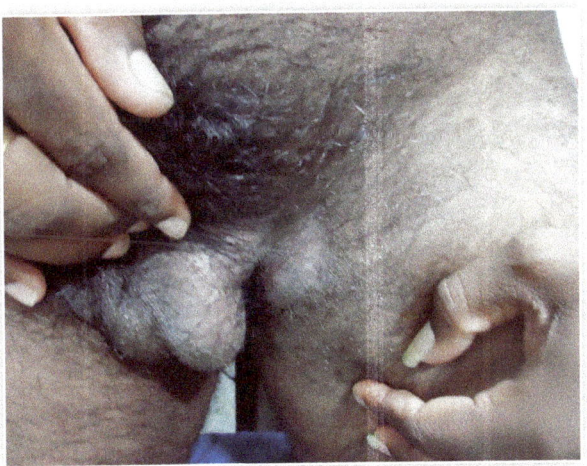

FIG. 48: Same patient as in figure 47.

Color Atlas of Dermatophytoses: *Focus on Superficial Fungal Infections*

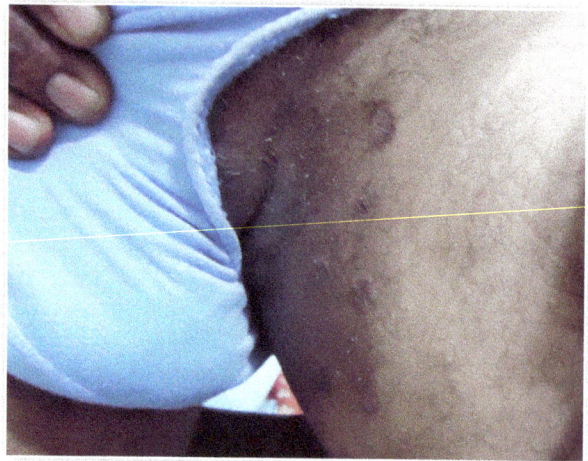

FIG. 49: Multiple small erythematous scaly patches.

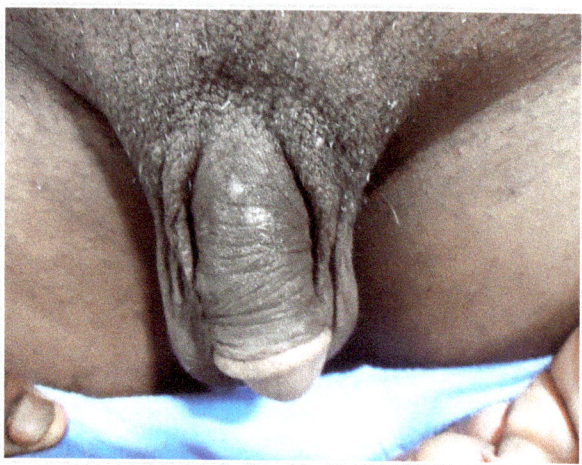

FIG. 50: Involvement of penile shaft.

Groin Infections

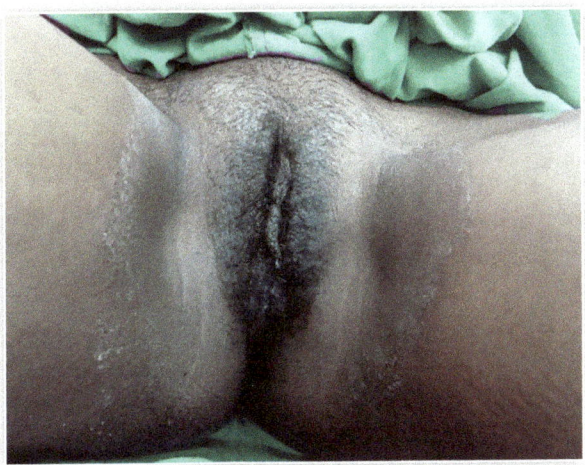

FIG. 51: Classical tinea cruris in a young girl.

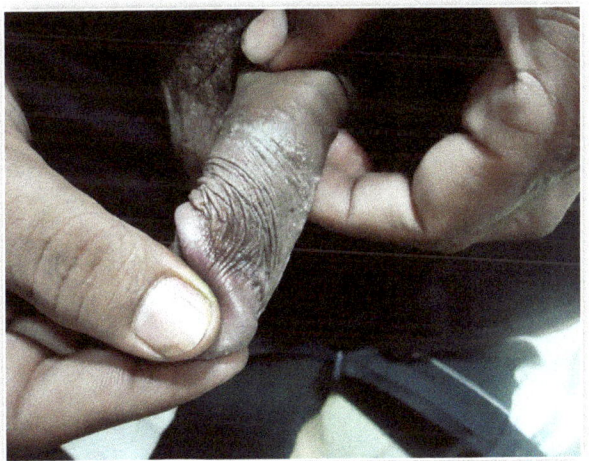

FIG. 52: Scaly patch over the penile shaft in addition to tinea cruris.

Color Atlas of Dermatophytoses: *Focus on Superficial Fungal Infections*

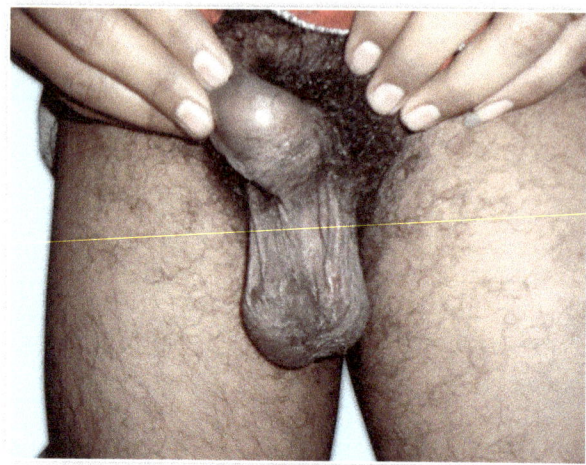

FIG. 53: Involvement of the scrotal skin posing difficulty in diagnosis.

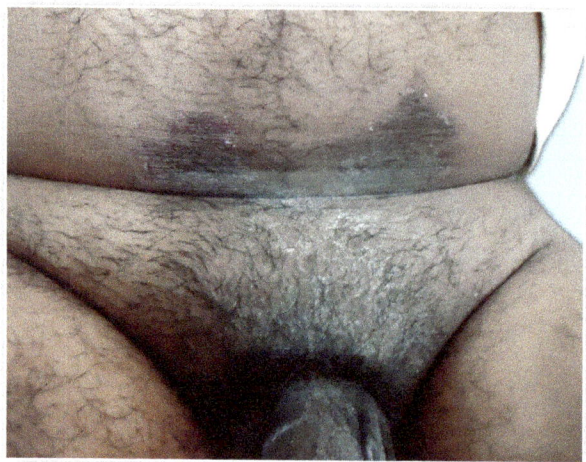

FIG. 54: Active margin over the lower abdomen.

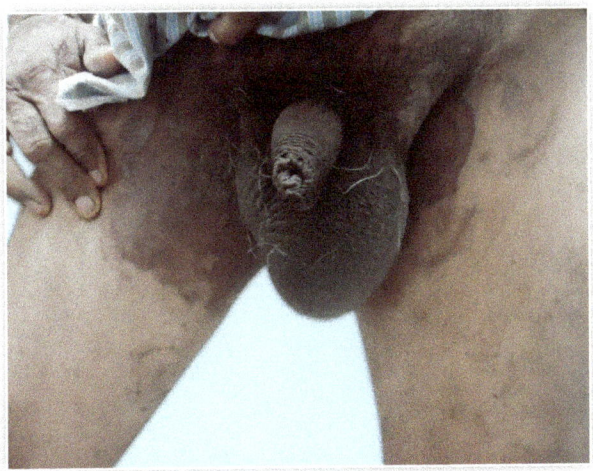

FIG. 55: Hyperpigmentation following treatment.

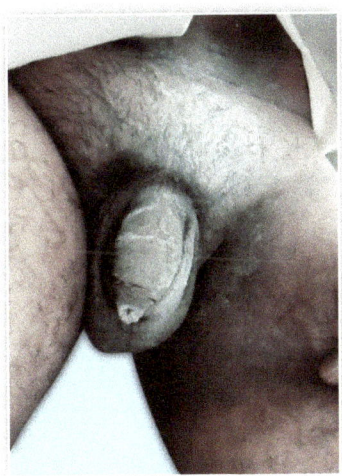

FIG. 56: Tinea genitalis, note the lichenification over the patch.

Color Atlas of Dermatophytoses: *Focus on Superficial Fungal Infections*

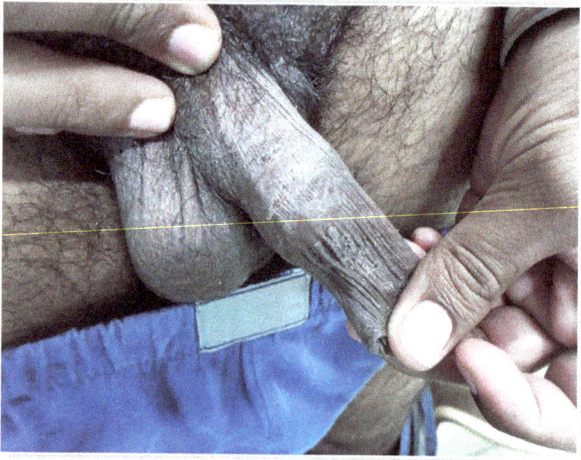

FIG. 57: Involvement of the penile shaft.

CHAPTER 7: Gluteal Area Infections

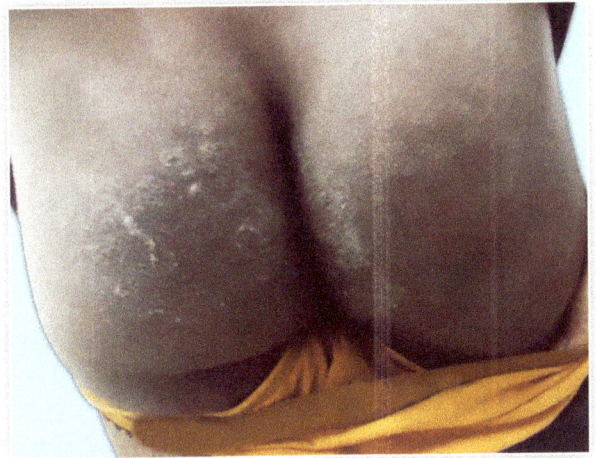

FIG. 1: Gluteal infection.

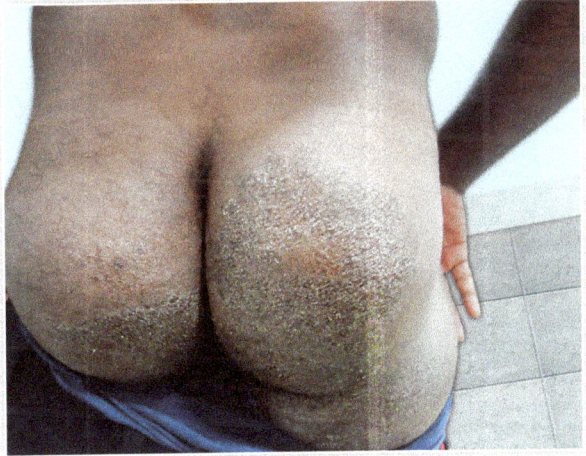

FIG. 2: Tinea glutealis showing central clearance over the right buttock.

Color Atlas of Dermatophytoses: *Focus on Superficial Fungal Infections*

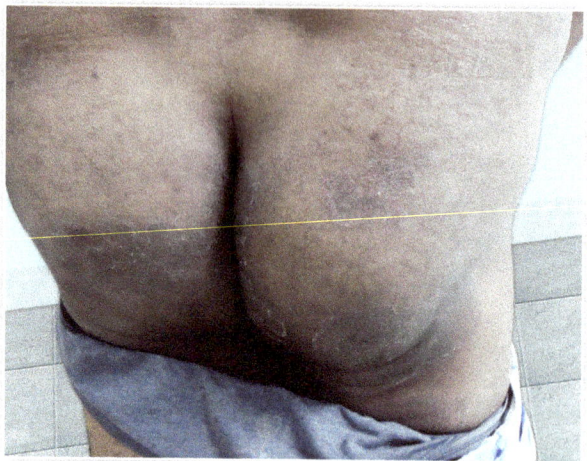

FIG. 3: Multiple small patches of tinea in the gluteal area.

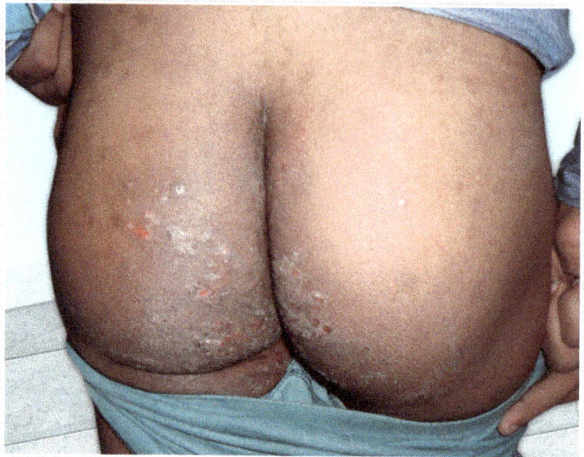

FIG. 4: Multiple excoriation marks in tinea glutealis.

Gluteal Area Infections

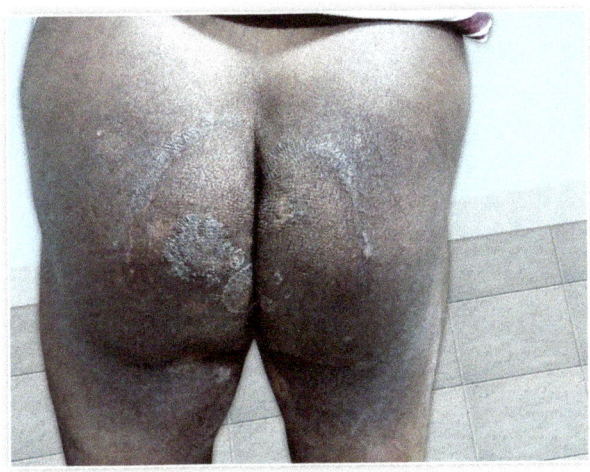

FIG. 5: Active margin and new patch appearing inside the patch.

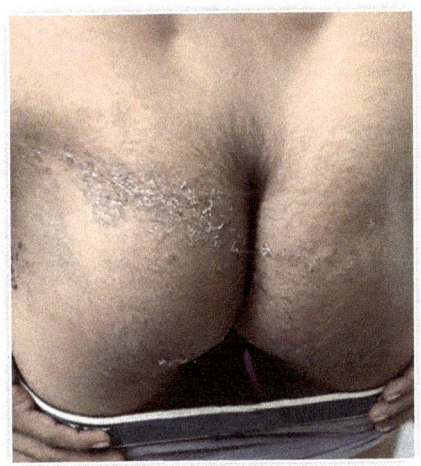

FIG. 6: Partially treated tinea glutealis having an irregular shape.

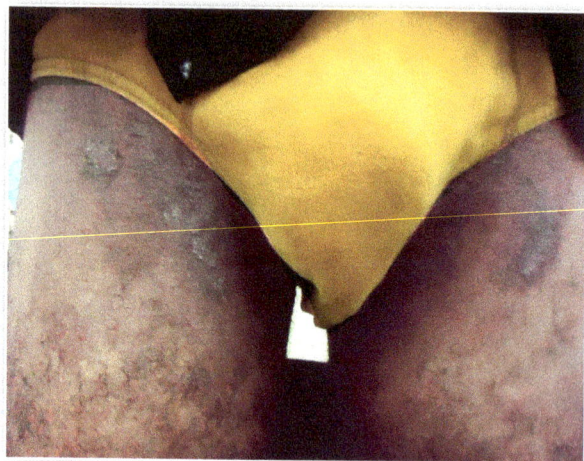

FIG. 7: Patient seen in figure 1. Note that gluteal infection spreads to crural area.

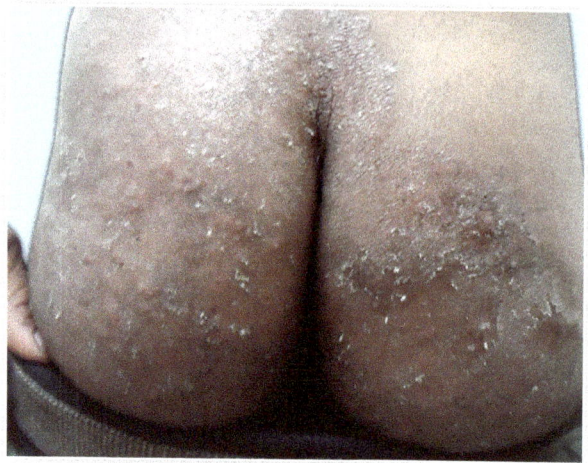

FIG. 8: Inflammatory type of tinea glutealis.

Gluteal Area Infections

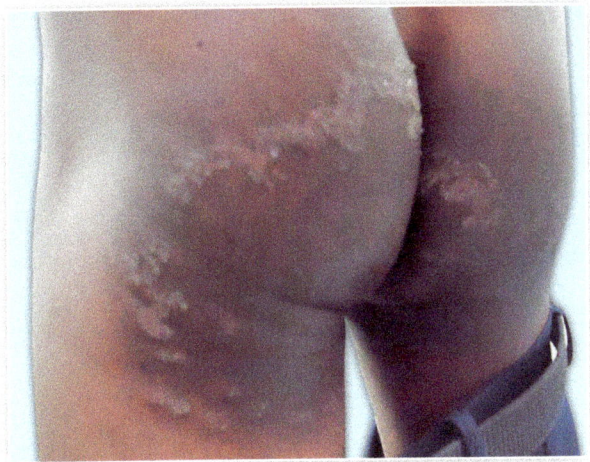

FIG. 9: Gluteal infection with active border.

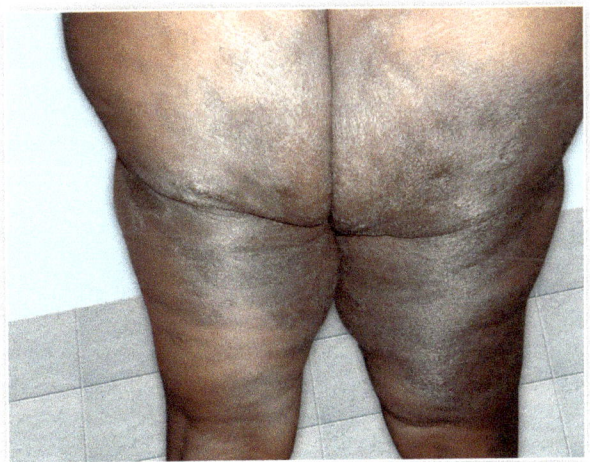

FIG. 10: Extensive tinea glutealis in a hypothyroid woman.

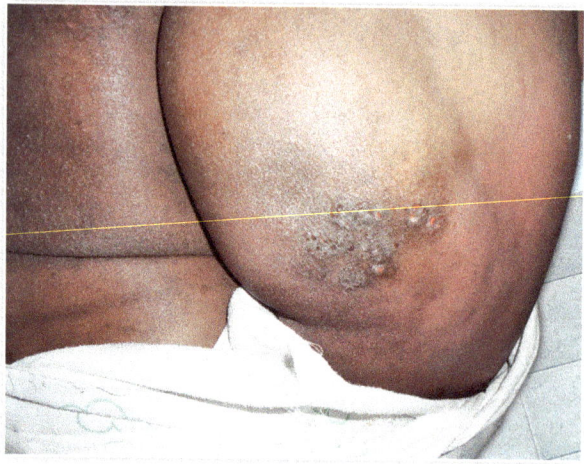

FIG. 11: Single patch of tinea glutealis.

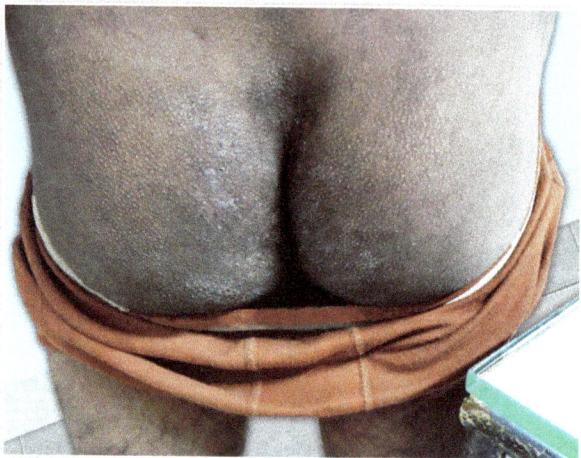

FIG. 12: Partially treated tinea glutealis showing irregular patch.

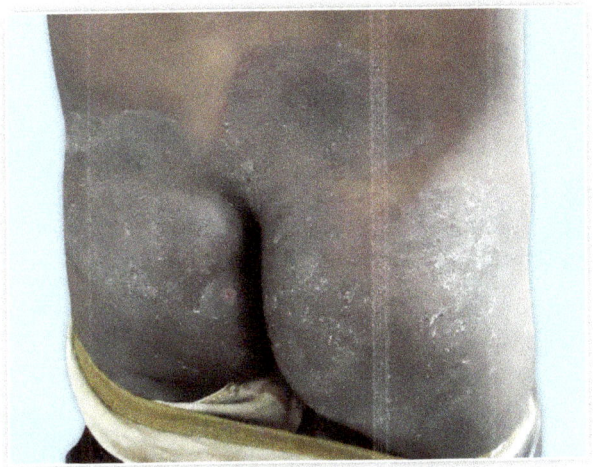

FIG. 13: Noninflammatory type of tinea glutealis.

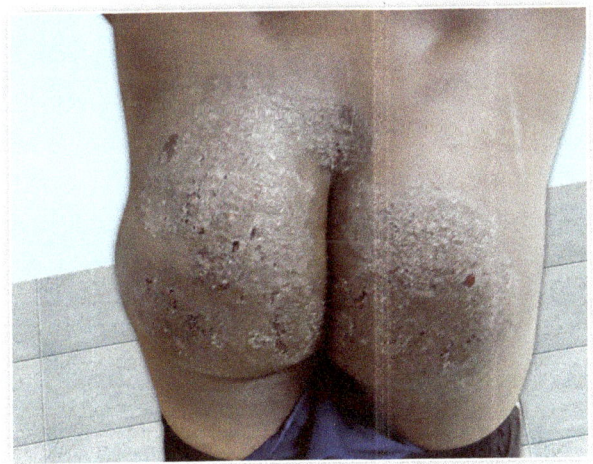

FIG. 14: Resistant tinea glutealis.

Color Atlas of Dermatophytoses: *Focus on Superficial Fungal Infections*

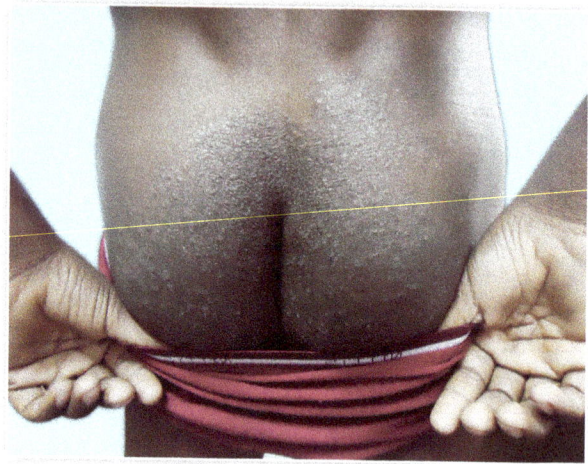

FIG. 15: Extensive involvement of tinea corporis in a hosteller.

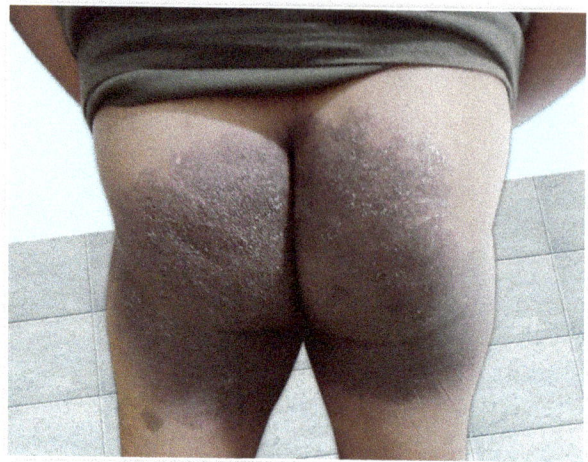

FIG. 16: Postinflammatory pigmentation with scaling.

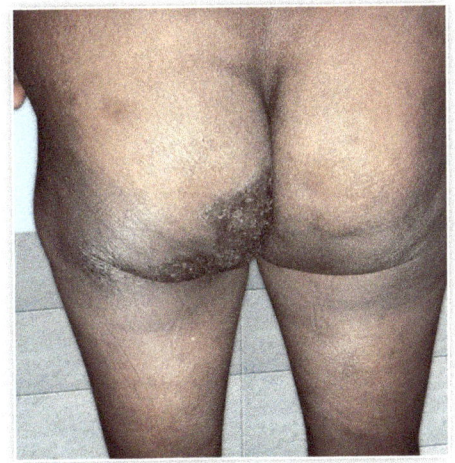

FIG. 17: Unilateral involvement.

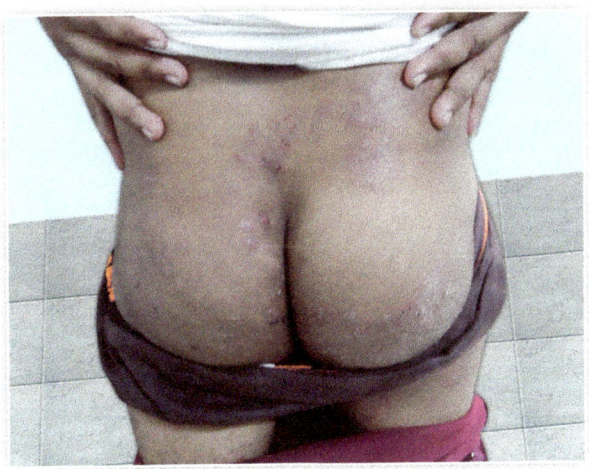

FIG. 18: Irregular patches of tinea glutealis.

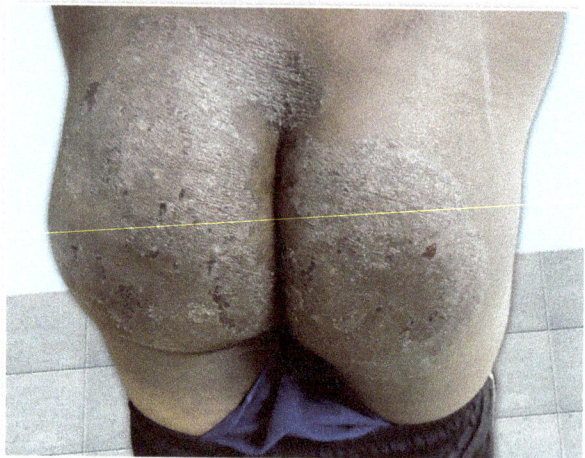

FIG. 19: Scaling of the entire patch without central clearance.

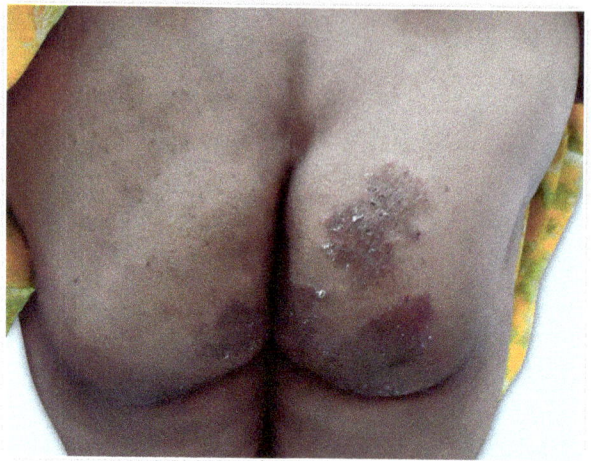

FIG. 20: Tinea glutealis with excoriation marks indicating intense itching.

Gluteal Area Infections

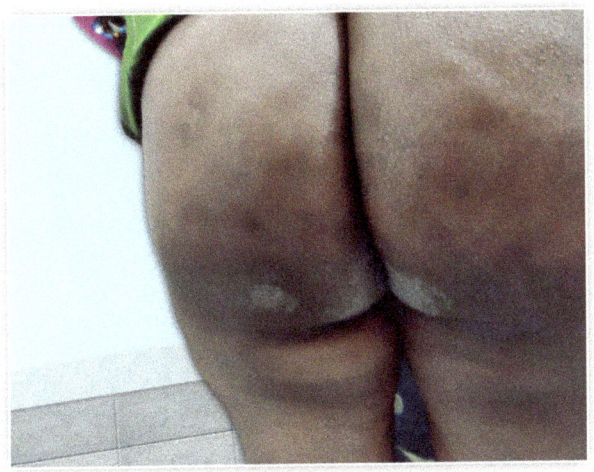

FIG. 21: Small patches which can be easily missed.

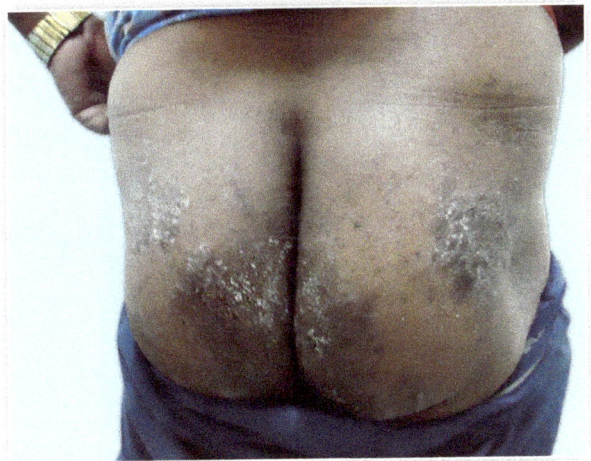

FIG. 22: Post-treatment pigmentation in case with recurrence.

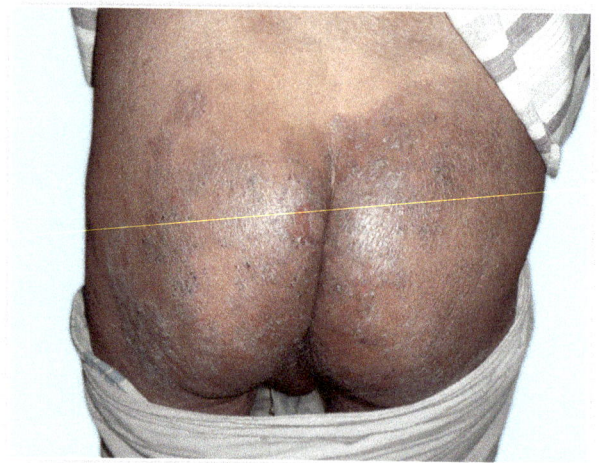

FIG. 23: Tinea glutealis in a hypothyroid patient, note the dry skin.

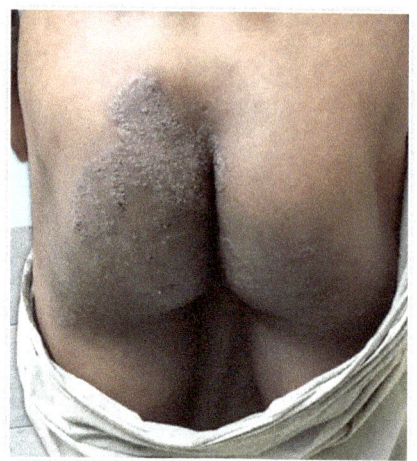

FIG. 24: Classical advancing border.

Gluteal Area Infections

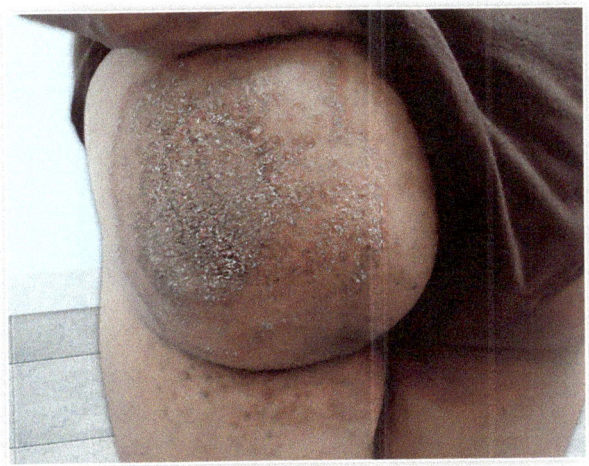

FIG. 25: Appearance of new patch and active advancing margin.

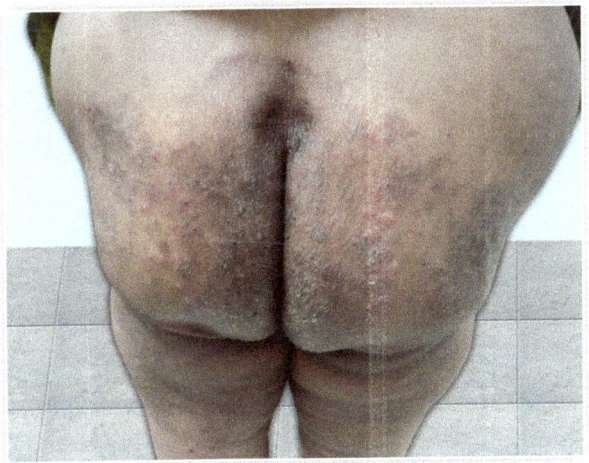

FIG. 26: Partially treated gluteal infection. Note the concentric nature.

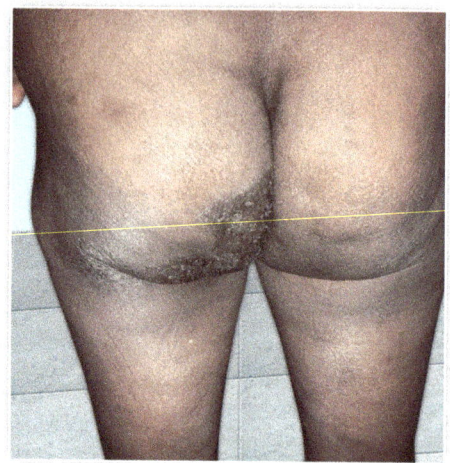

FIG. 27: Tinea glutealis affecting only one side.

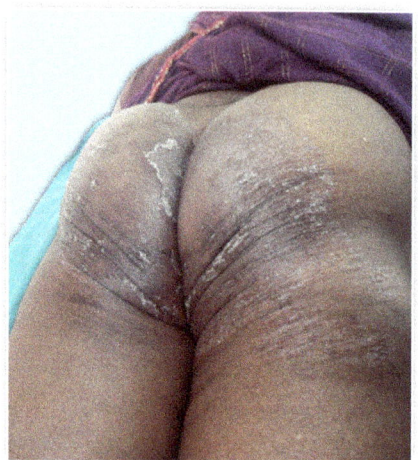

FIG. 28: Noninflammatory type of tinea glutealis.

Gluteal Area Infections

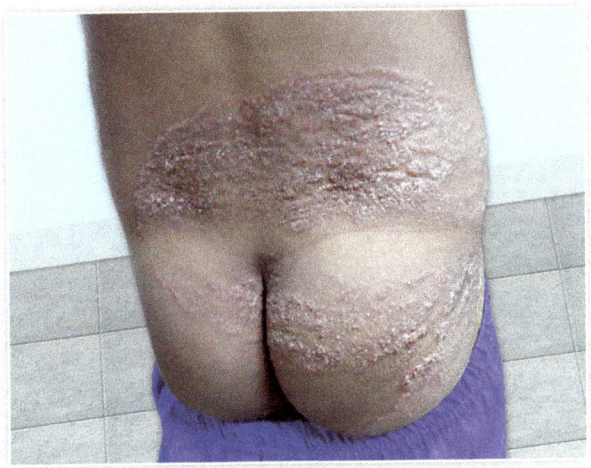

FIG. 29: Big patch with central clearance.

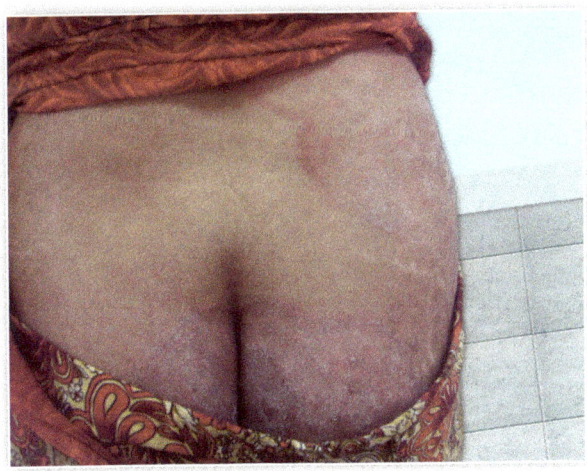

FIG. 30: Tinea glutealis in a patient with tinea corporis.

Color Atlas of Dermatophytoses: *Focus on Superficial Fungal Infections*

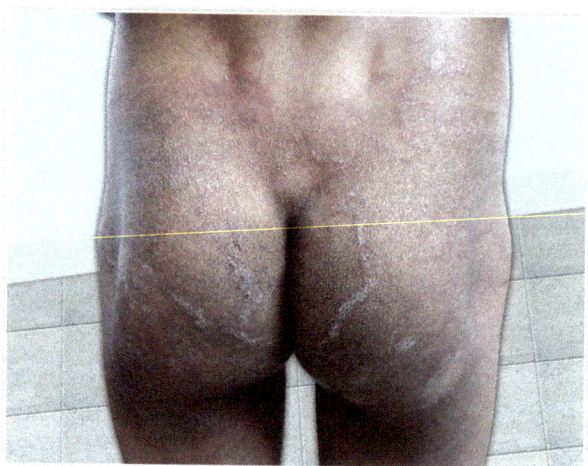

FIG. 31: Persisting margin even after a full course of treatment.

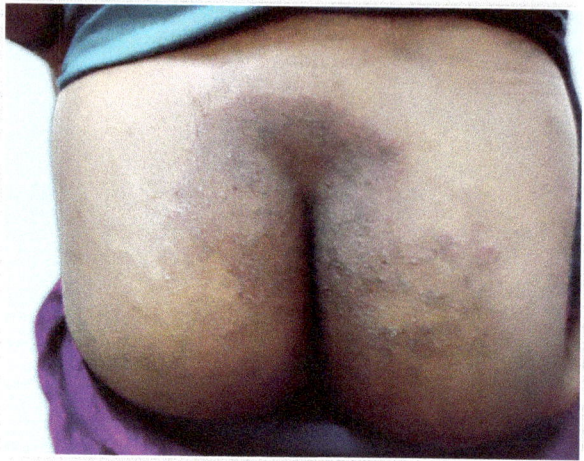

FIG. 32: Ill-defined patch can be easily missed in a dark individual.

Gluteal Area Infections

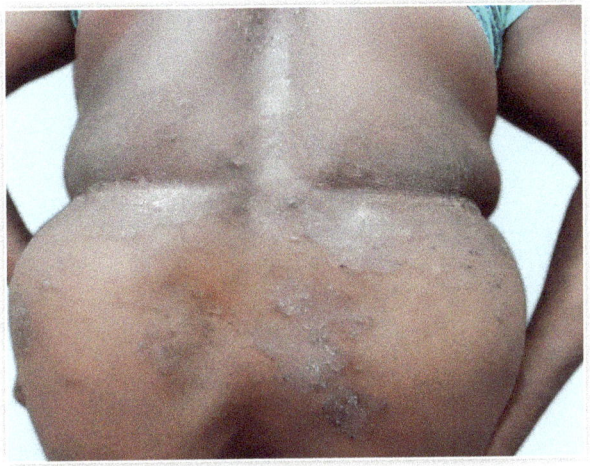

FIG. 33: Infection spreading from trunk to gluteal region.

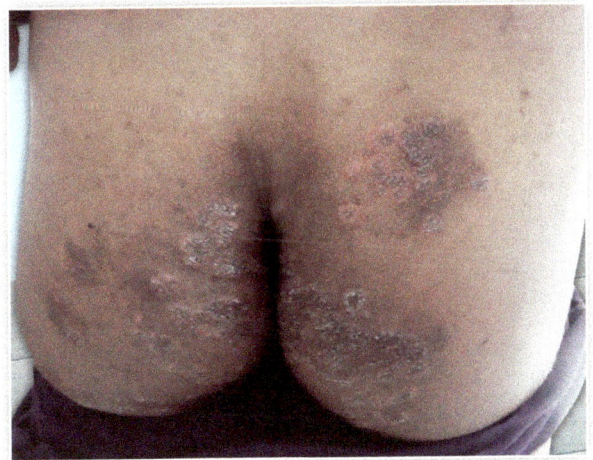

FIG. 34: Multiple small patches coalescing to form larger patches.

Color Atlas of Dermatophytoses: *Focus on Superficial Fungal Infections*

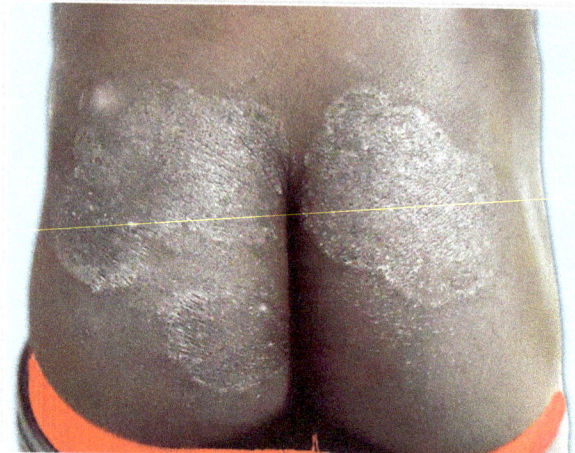

FIG. 35: Active patches in a boy.

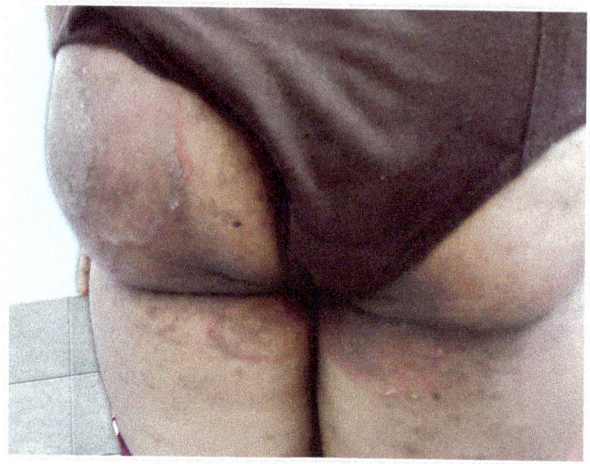

FIG. 36: Resistant tinea glutealis that frequently recurred.

Gluteal Area Infections

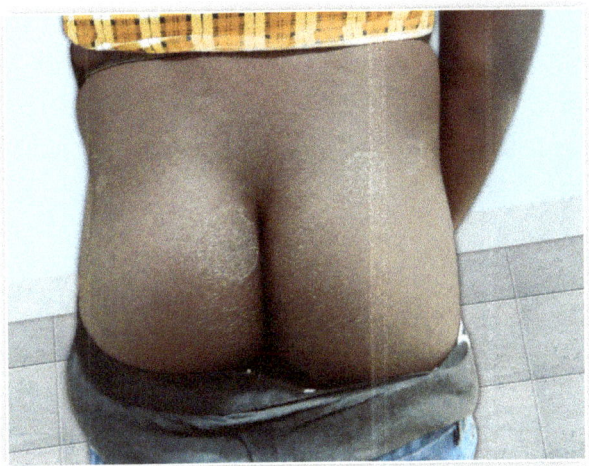

FIG. 37: Multiple patches in a boy.

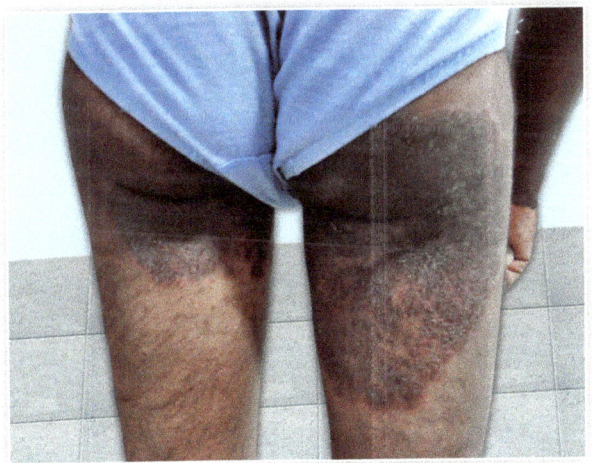

FIG. 38: Extension on to the thigh in a patient (driver).

Color Atlas of Dermatophytoses: *Focus on Superficial Fungal Infections*

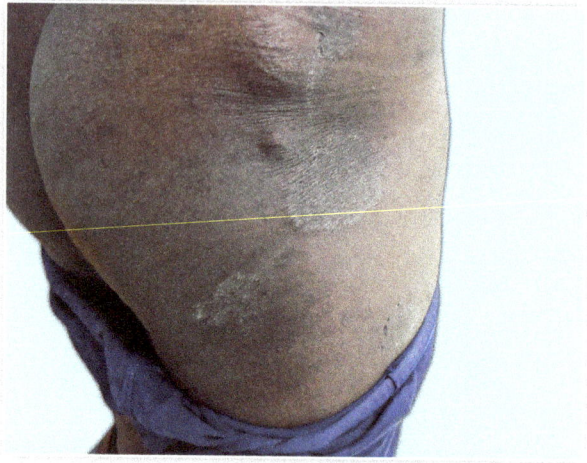

FIG. 39: Tinea corporis spilling over to gluteal area.

CHAPTER 8: Feet Infections

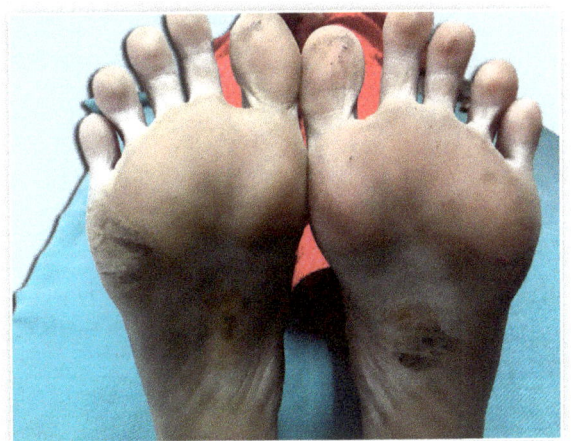

FIG. 1: Unilateral scaly plaque mimicking psoriasis ped.

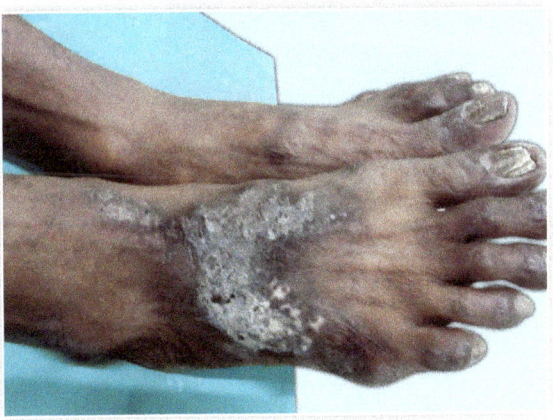

FIG. 2: Unilateral scaly plaque of dermatophytosis of foot mimicking psoriasis.

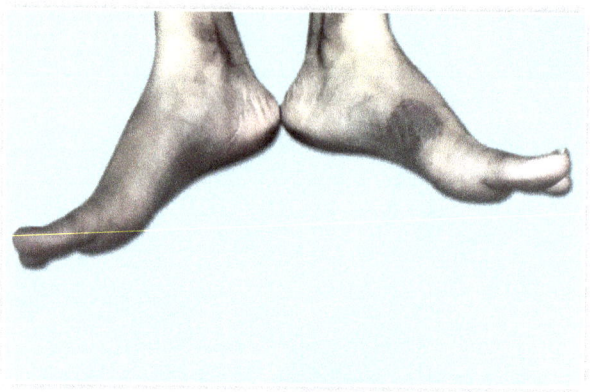

FIG. 3: Hyperpigmentation following treatment with irritant.

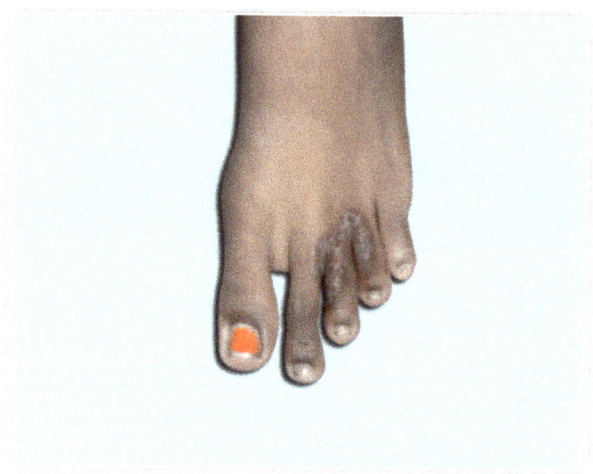

FIG. 4: Tinea pedis mimicking psoriasis.

Feet Infections

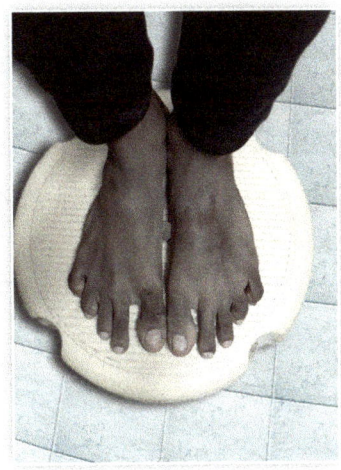

FIG. 5: Tinea pedes, note the unilateral affection.

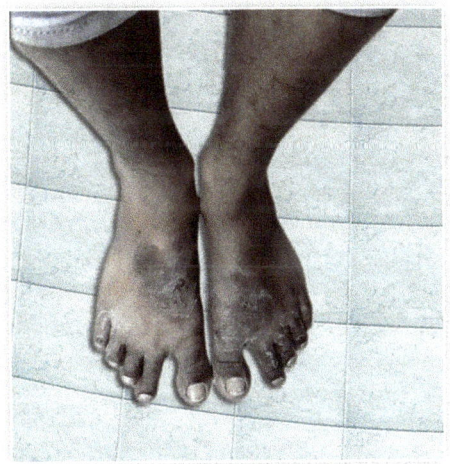

FIG. 6: Bilateral involvement not uncommon in tinea pedes.

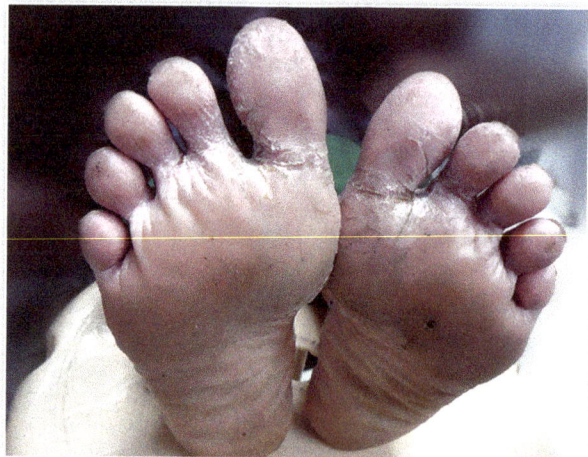

FIG. 7: Bilateral tinea pedes treated as eczema for long.

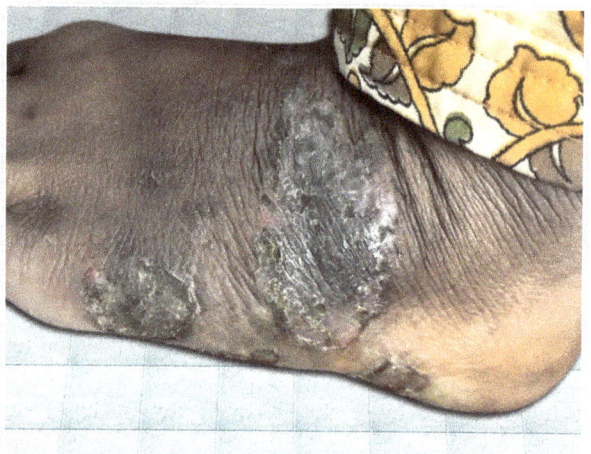

FIG. 8: Tenia pedes in a diabetic patient.

Feet Infections

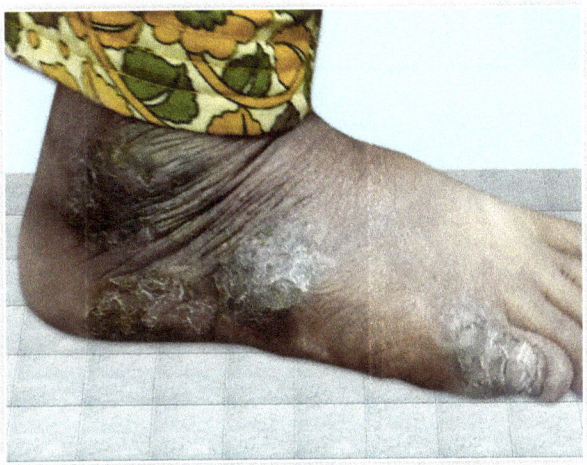

FIG. 9: Same patient as in figure 8.

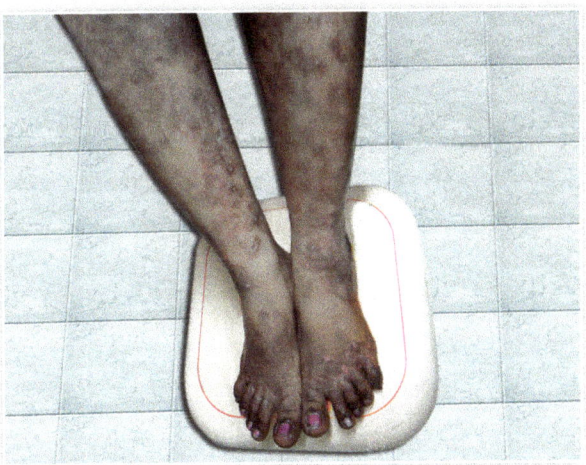

FIG. 10: Involvement of both feet in an atopic, note the well-defined margin.

CHAPTER 9: Nail Infections

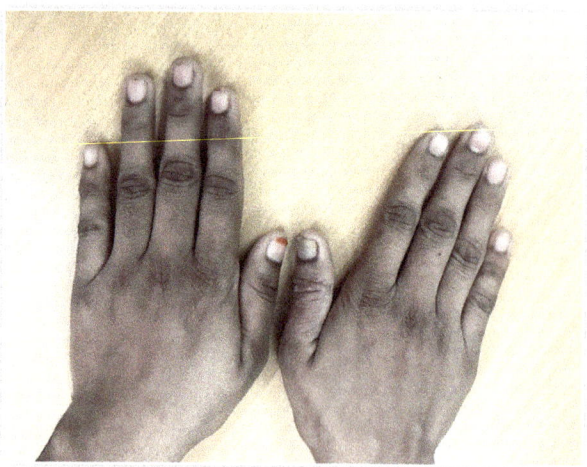

FIG. 1: Involvement of left thumbnail. Note involvement of nearby skin.

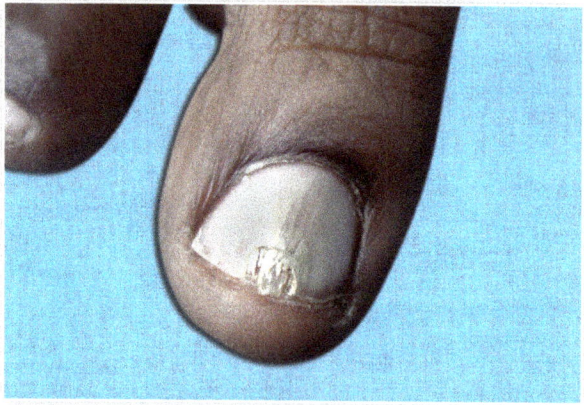

FIG. 2: Tinea unguium—white superficial onychomycosis.

Nail Infections

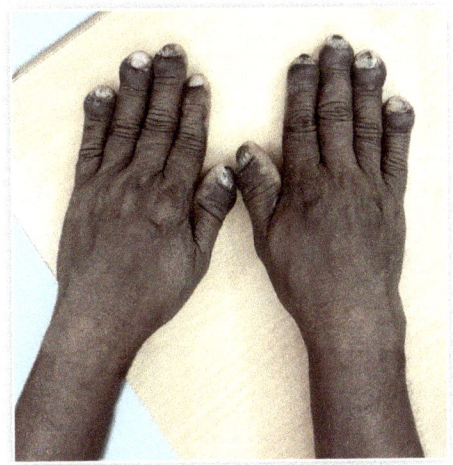

FIG. 3: Tinea unguium in an agricultural worker.

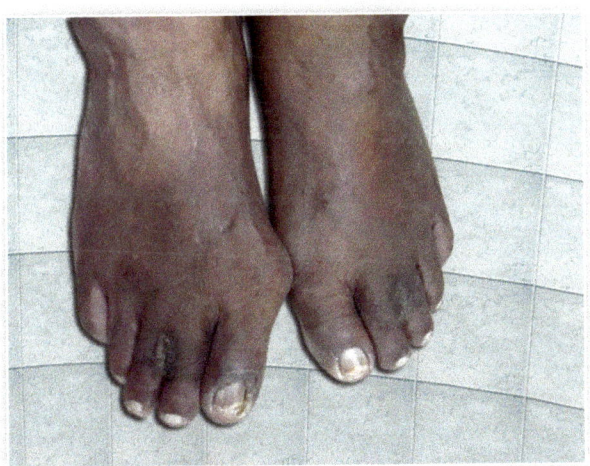

FIG. 4: Tinea unguium of the right big toe nail with intertrigo.

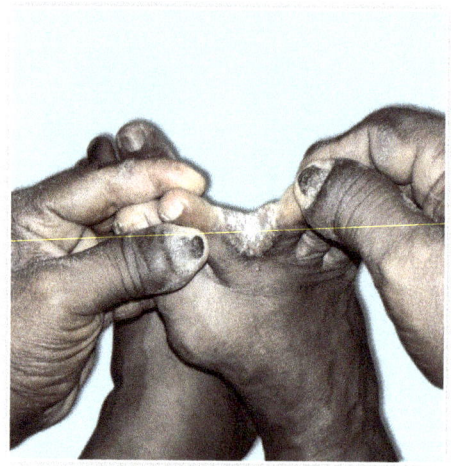

FIG. 5: Same patient as in figure 4.

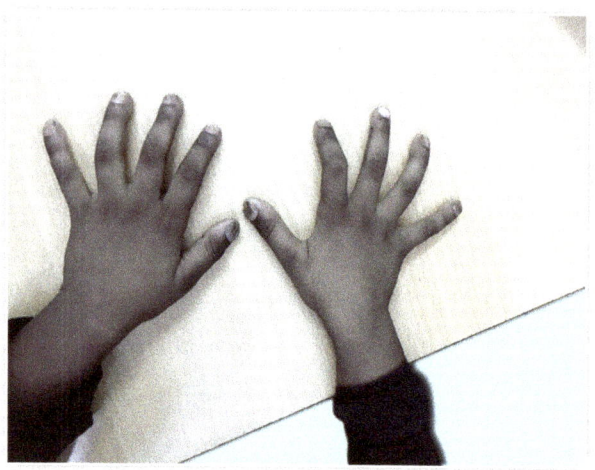

FIG. 6: Tinea unguium, note bilateral but asymmetric involvement.

Nail Infections

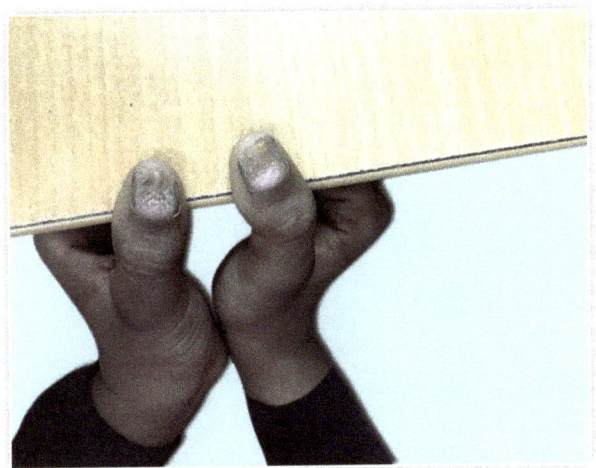

FIG. 7: Same patient as in figure 6.

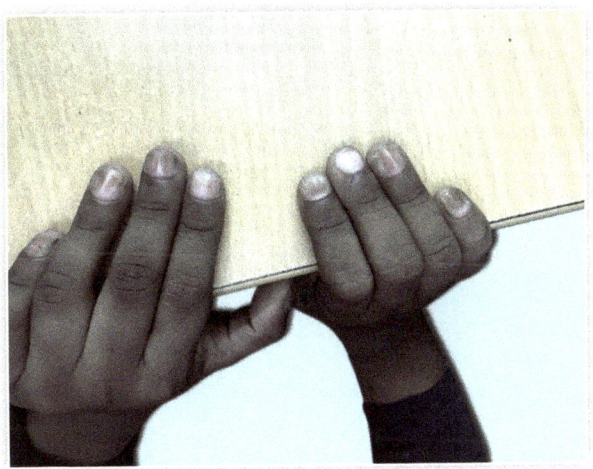

FIG. 8: Same patient as in figure 6.

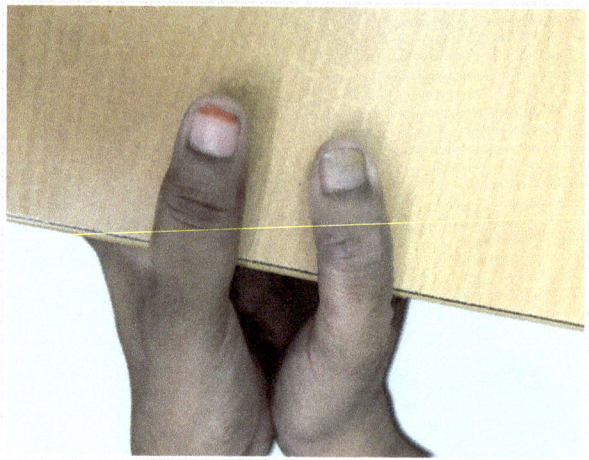

FIG. 9: Onychomycosis of right thumb.

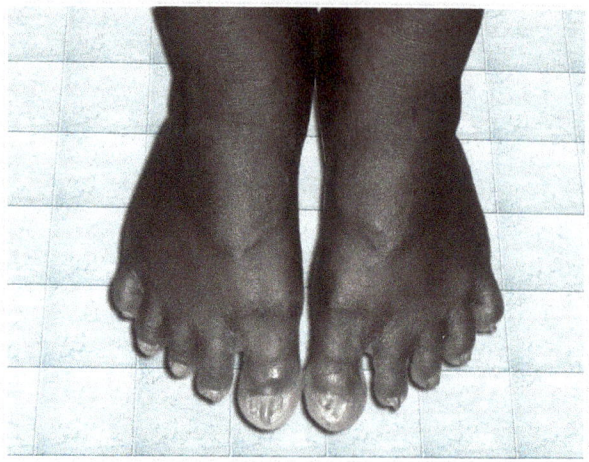

FIG. 10: Tinea unguium in an agricultural worker.

CHAPTER 10: Steroid-modified Disease

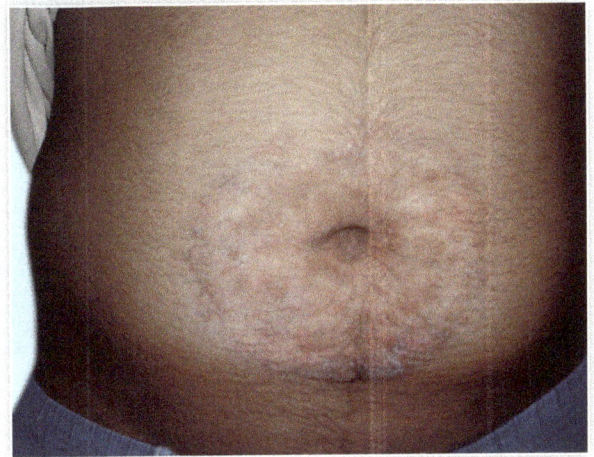

FIG. 1: Topical steroid modified tinea corporis showing ring within ring.

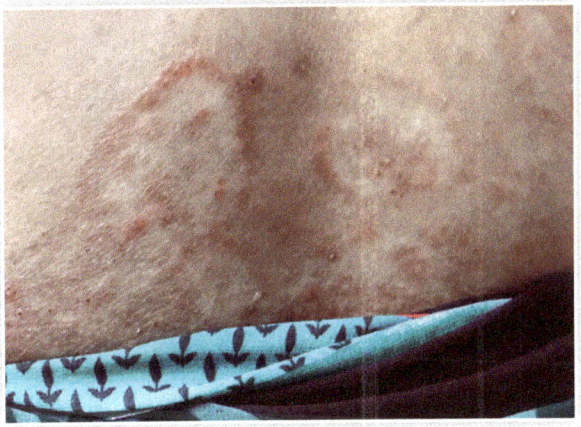

FIG. 2: Steroid-modified tinea corporis still showing active margin.

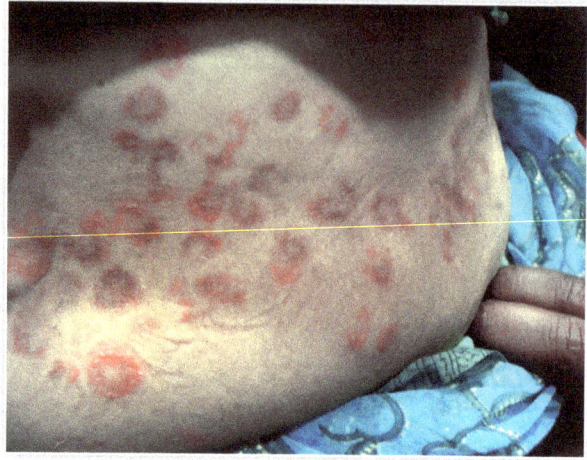

FIG. 3: Steroid-modified tinea corporis.

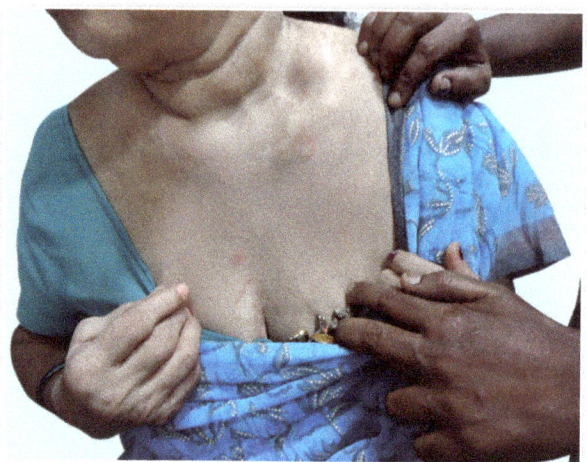

FIG. 4: Same patient as in figure 3.

Steroid-modified Disease

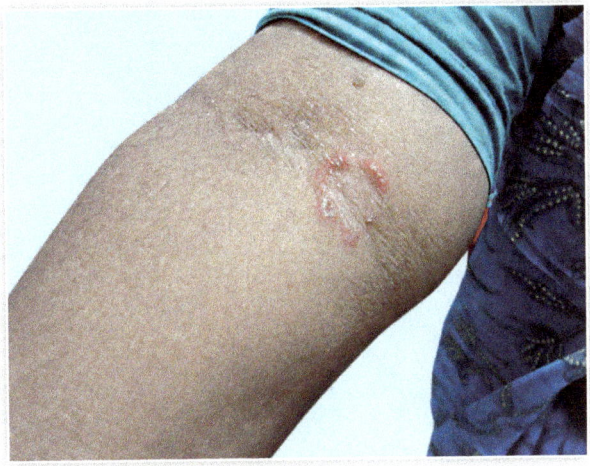

FIG. 5: Same patient as in figure 3.

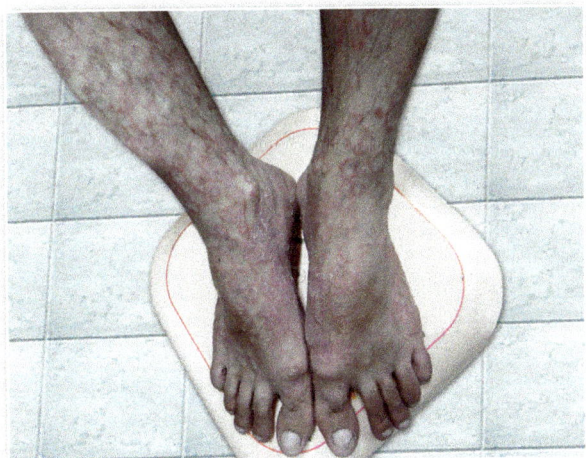

FIG. 6: Multiple patches following treatment with steroid combination.

Color Atlas of Dermatophytoses: *Focus on Superficial Fungal Infections*

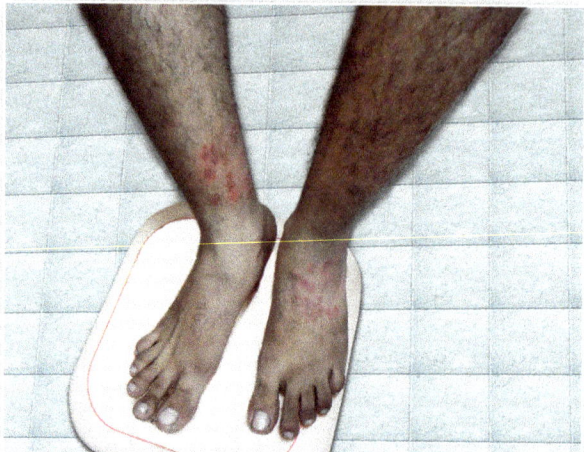

FIG. 7: The erythema and multiple lesions following steroid application.

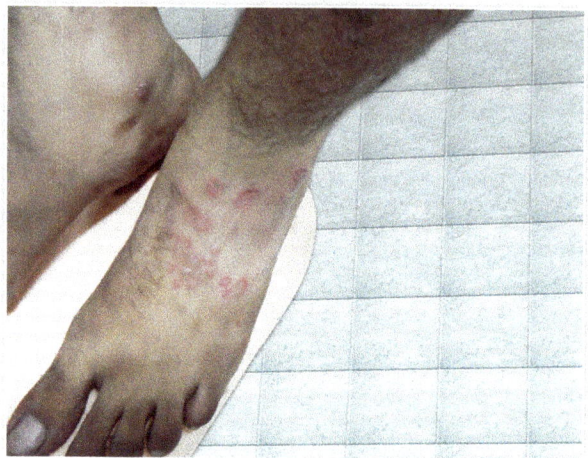

FIG. 8: Same patient as in figure 7.

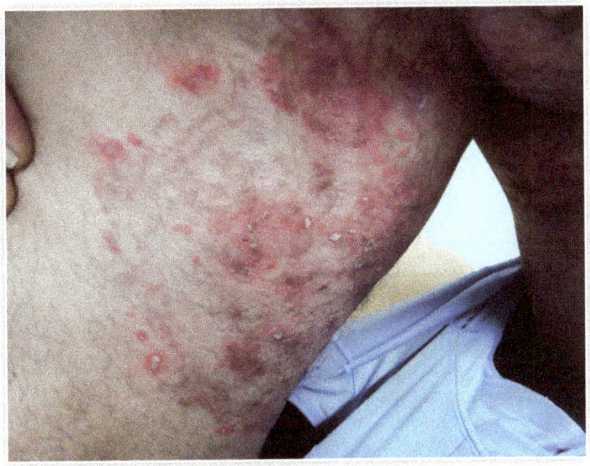

FIG. 9: Tinea cruris treated with topical steroid.

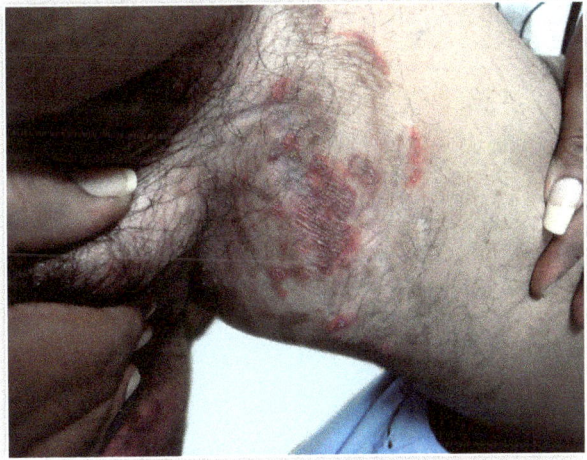

FIG. 10: Same patient as in figure 9, note the striae.

Color Atlas of Dermatophytoses: *Focus on Superficial Fungal Infections*

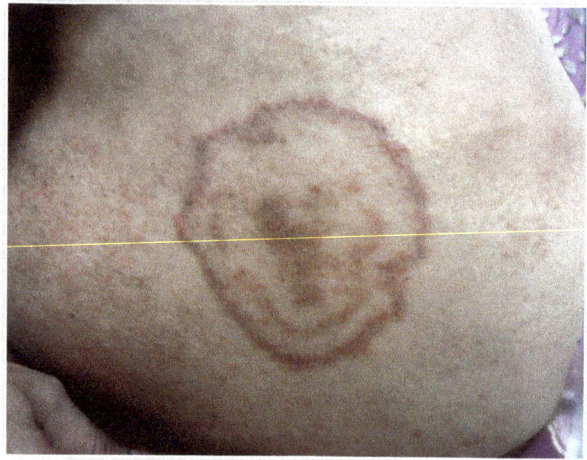

FIG. 11: Recurrence following topical steroid application.

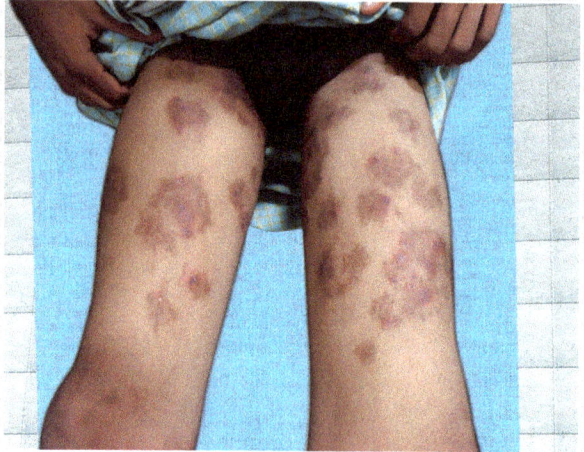

FIG. 12: Steroid-modified dermatophytosis.

Steroid-modified Disease

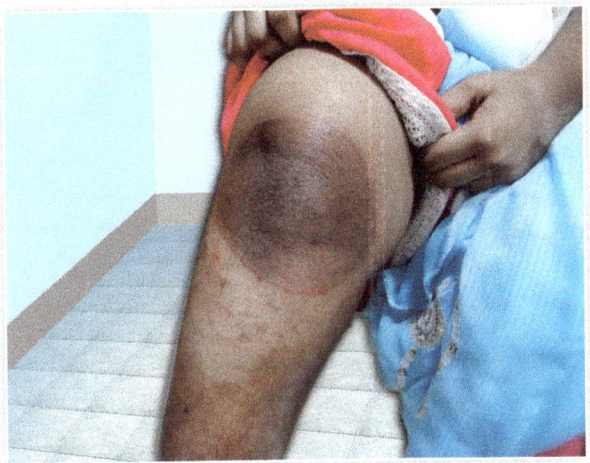

FIG. 13: Worsening following topical steroid therapy.

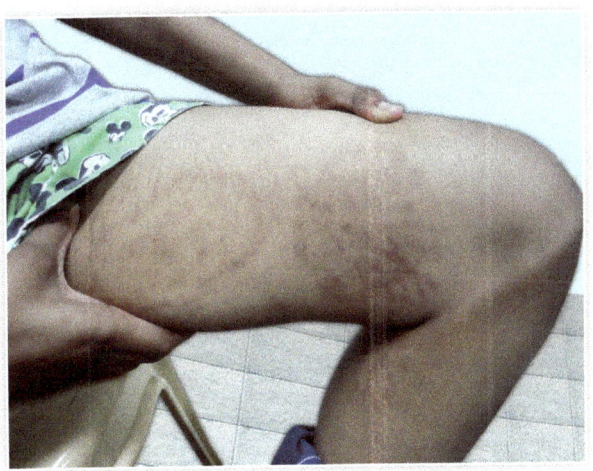

FIG. 14: Note the striae as a result of steroid application.

Color Atlas of Dermatophytoses: *Focus on Superficial Fungal Infections*

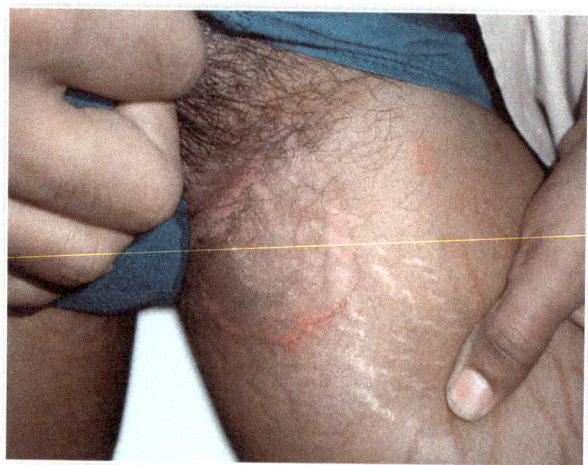

FIG. 15: Same patient as in figure 14.

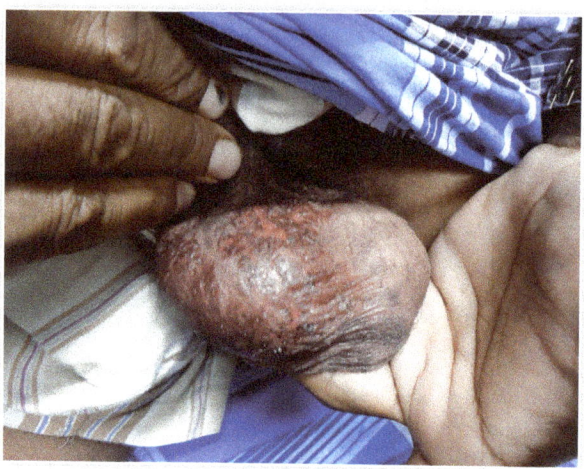

FIG. 16: Irritant reaction following salicylic acid combination.

Steroid-modified Disease

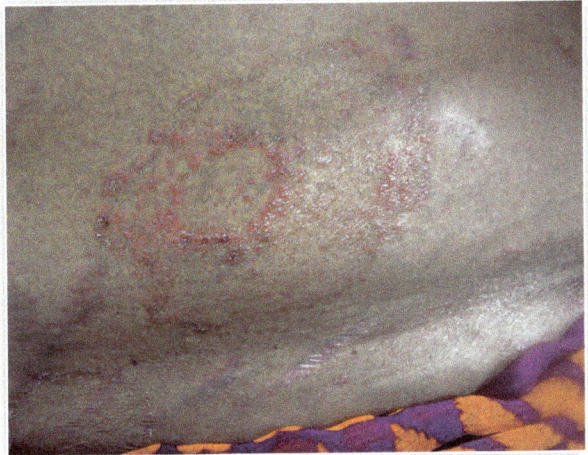

FIG. 17: New patch with central clearance while on topical steroid therapy.

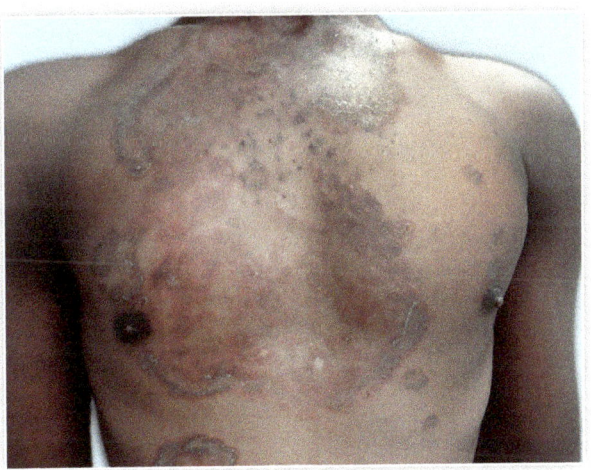

FIG. 18: Steroid-modified extensive dermatophytosis.

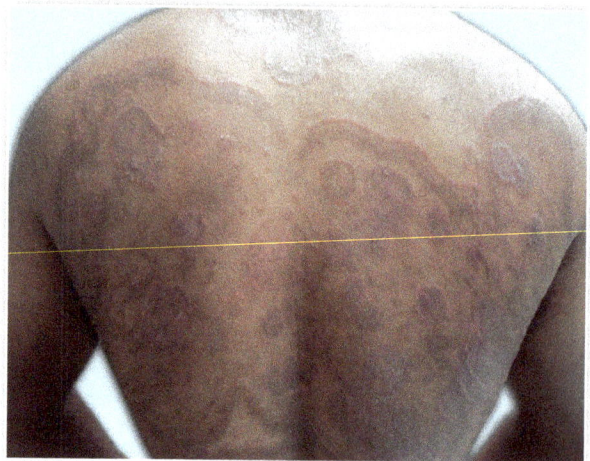

FIG. 19: Same patient as in figure 18.

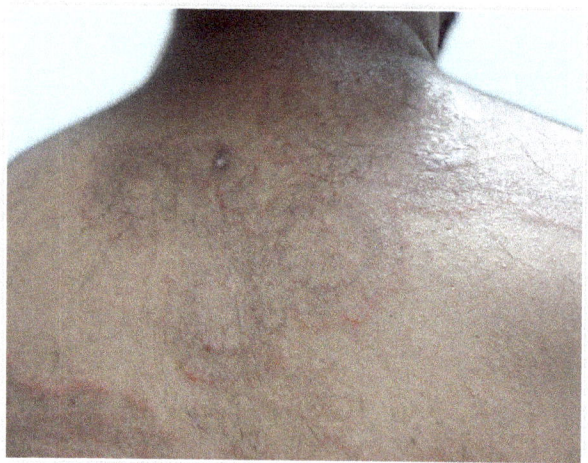

FIG. 20: Same patient as in figure 19.

Steroid-modified Disease

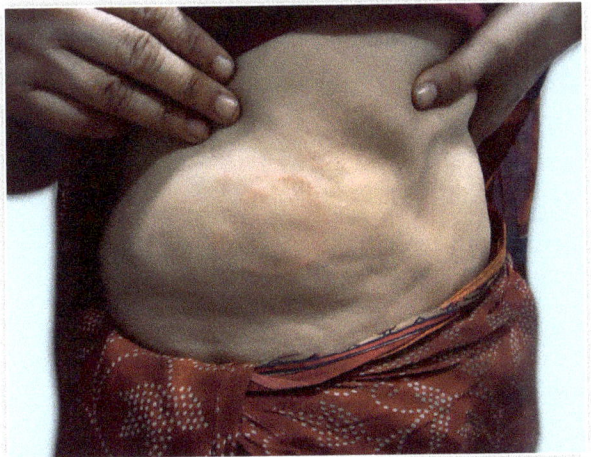

FIG. 21: Steroid-modified tinea corporis, note only the erythematous margin.

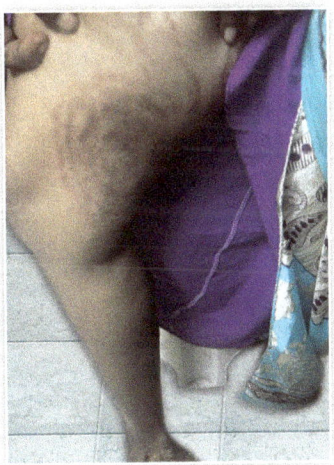

FIG. 22: The ring within ring appearance well seen after treatment.

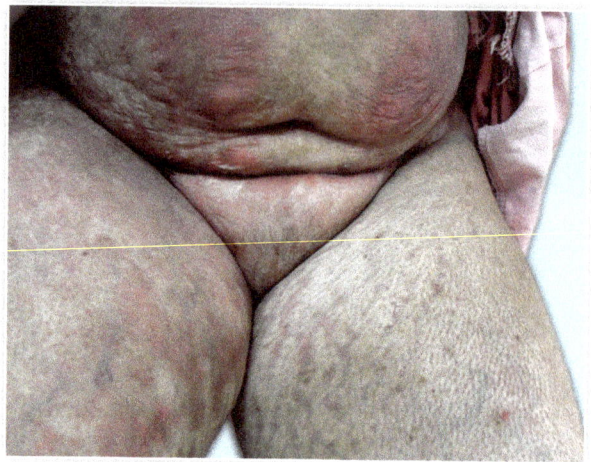

FIG. 23: Extensive striae following topical steroid treatment.

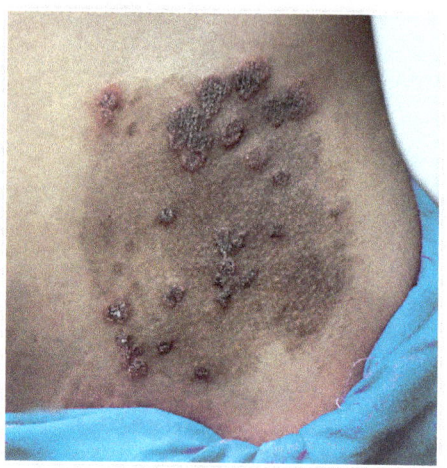

FIG. 24: Multiple small patches soon after stopping topical steroid.

Steroid-modified Disease

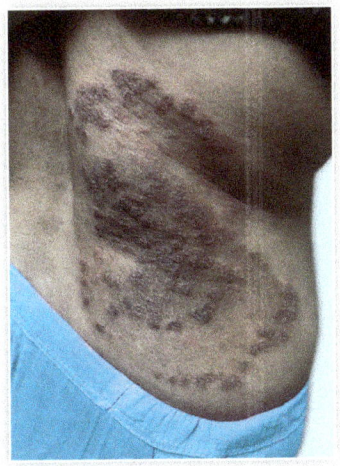

FIG. 25: Same patient as in figure 24.

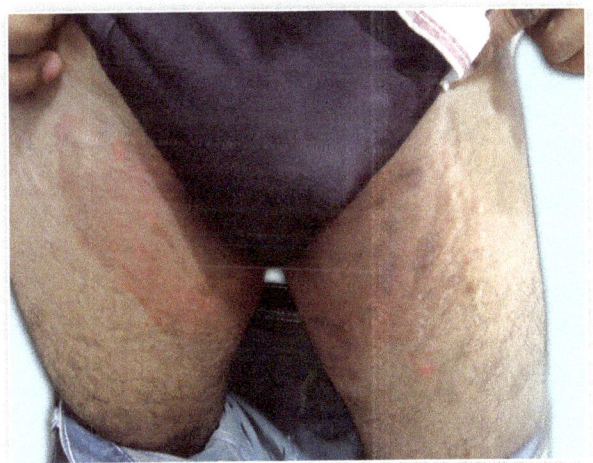

FIG. 26: The striae as a result of topical steroid combination.

Color Atlas of Dermatophytoses: *Focus on Superficial Fungal Infections*

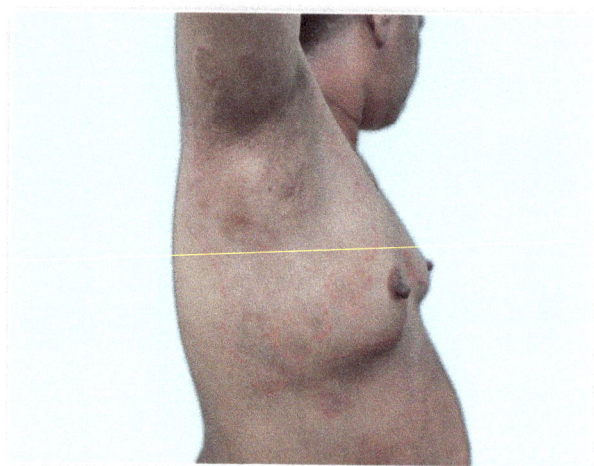

FIG. 27: Rapid extension of lesions following topical steroids.

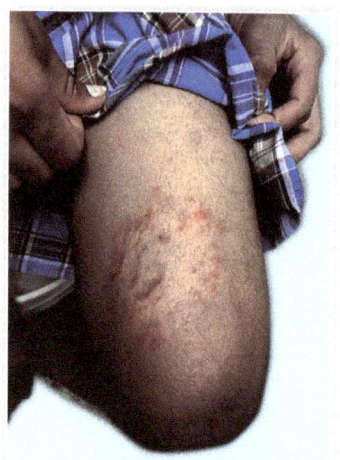

FIG. 28: Steroid-modified tinea corporis which has lost classical features.

Steroid-modified Disease

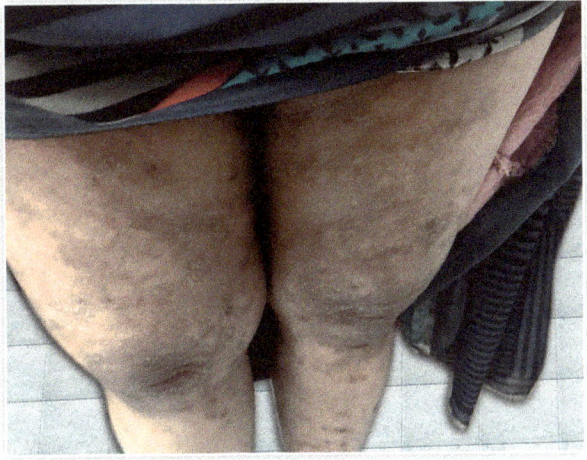

FIG. 29: Multiple patches mimicking pityriasis rosea following treatment.

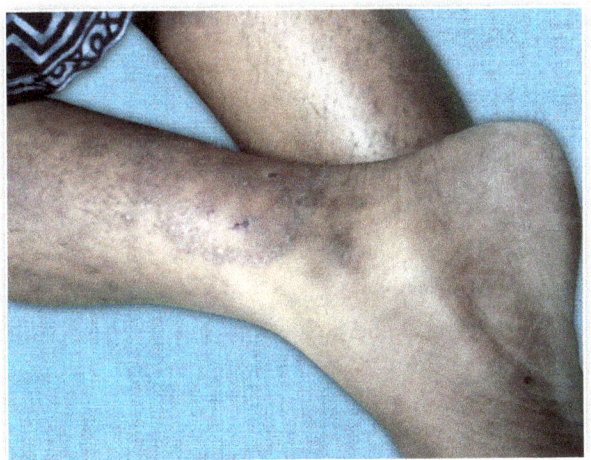

FIG. 30: Circle within circle with use of topical steroids in tinea infections.

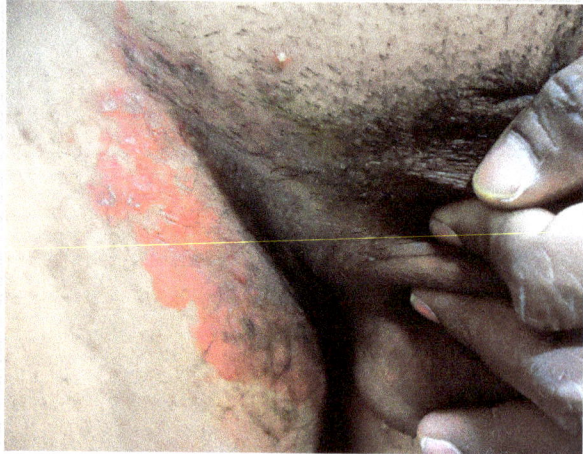

FIG. 31: Erythema and striae following topical steroid therapy.

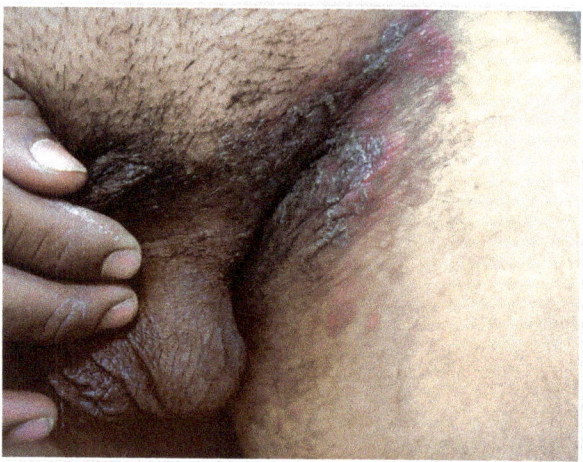

FIG. 32: Same patient as in figure 31.

Steroid-modified Disease

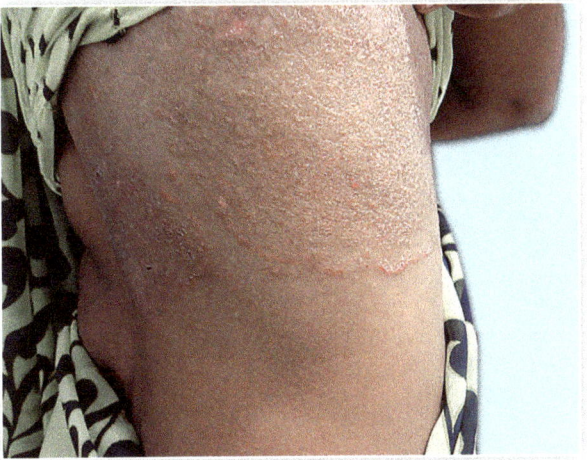

FIG. 33: Increase in size of lesion following steroid application.

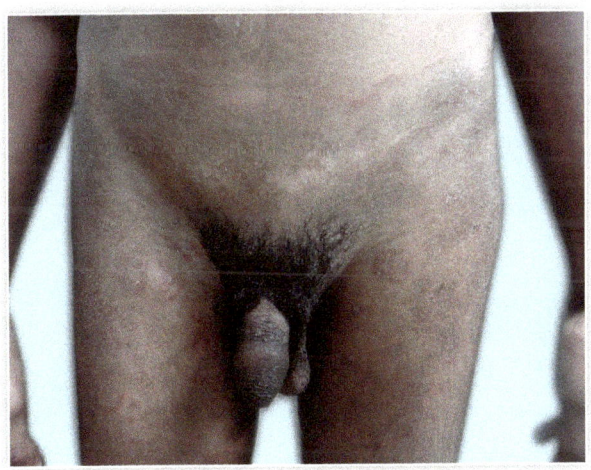

FIG. 34: Worsening of disease following topical steroid treatment.

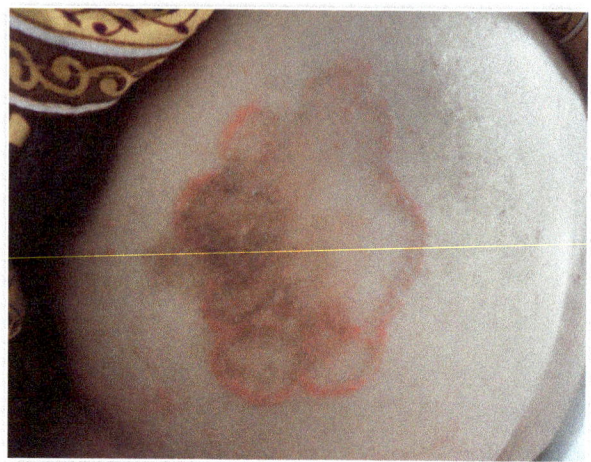

FIG. 35: A small patch mismanaged develops pustules.

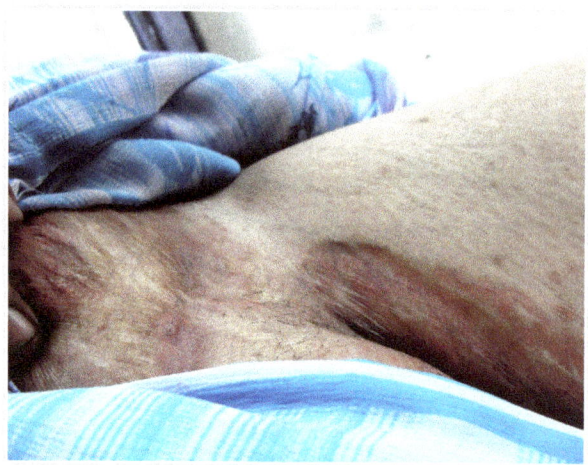

FIG. 36: Atrophy and striae following triple combination therapy.

Steroid-modified Disease

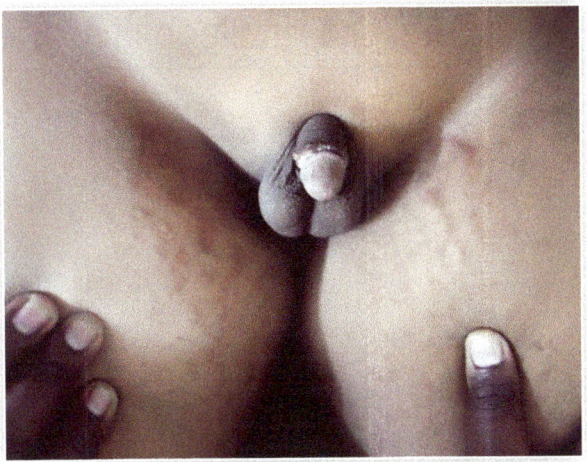

FIG. 37: Steroid combination leading to striae in a small boy.

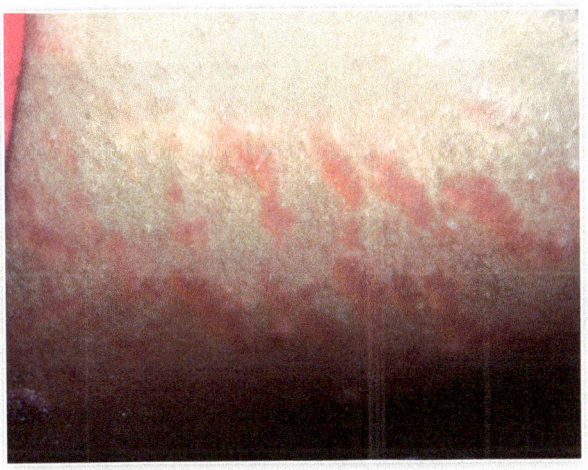

FIG. 38: Steroid damaged groin showing an active patch.

CHAPTER 11: Infections in Pregnancy

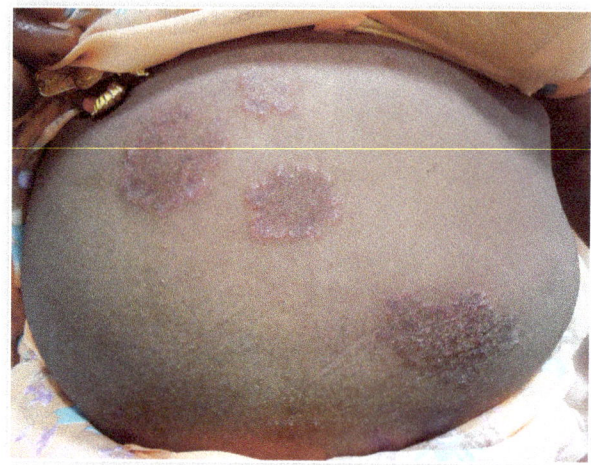

FIG. 1: Multiple patches of tinea corporis in pregnant woman.

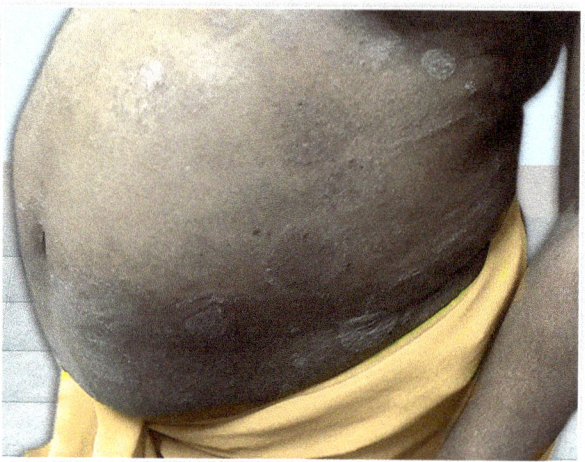

FIG. 2: Extensive tinea corporis in a pregnant lady, a therapeutic challenge.

Infections in Pregnancy

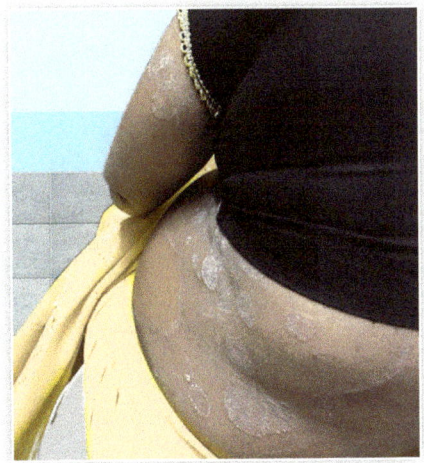

FIG. 3: Same patient as in figure 2.

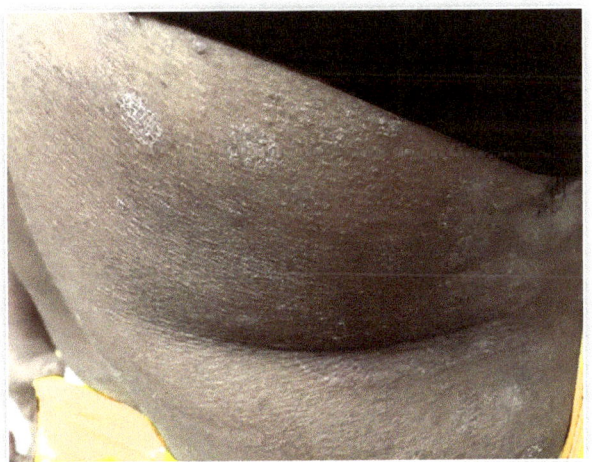

FIG. 4: Same patient as in figure 2.

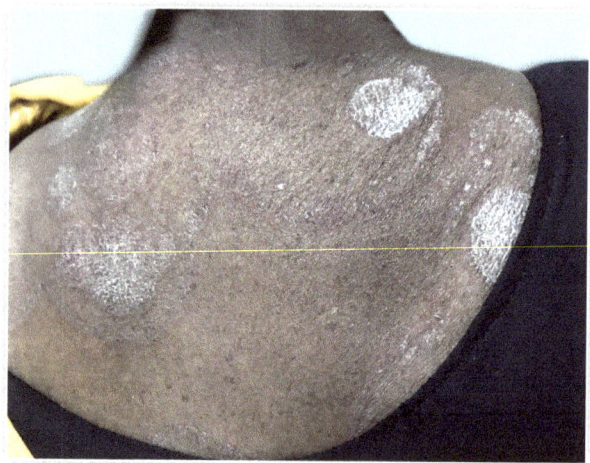

FIG. 5: Same patient as in figure 2.

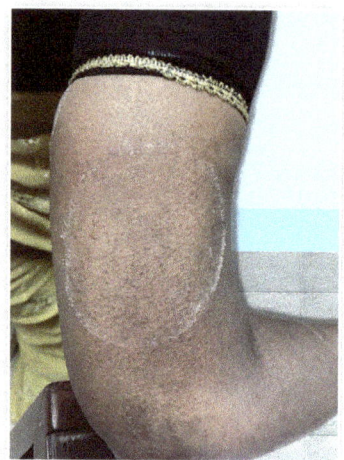

FIG. 6: Same patient as in figure 2.

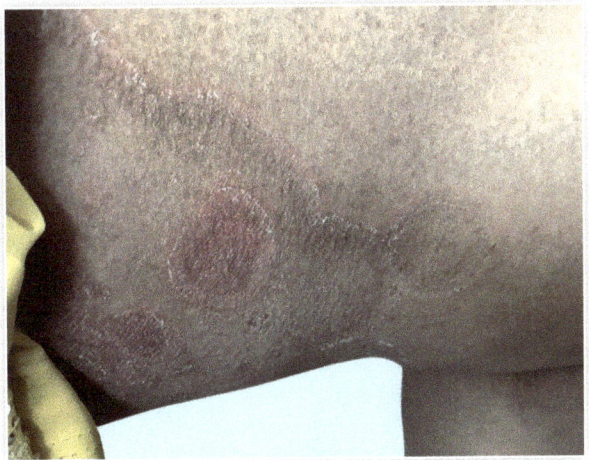

FIG. 7: Same patient as in figure 2.

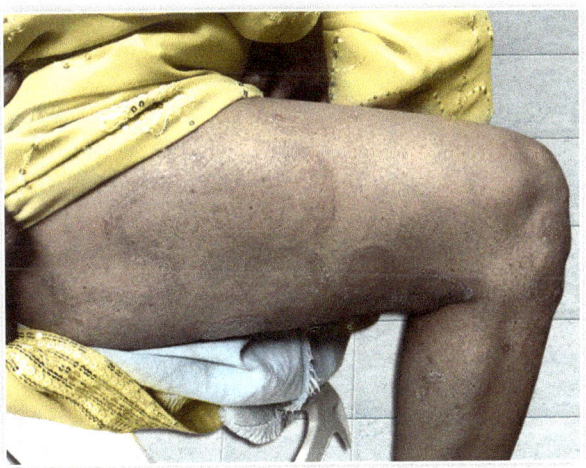

FIG. 8: Same patient as in figure 2.

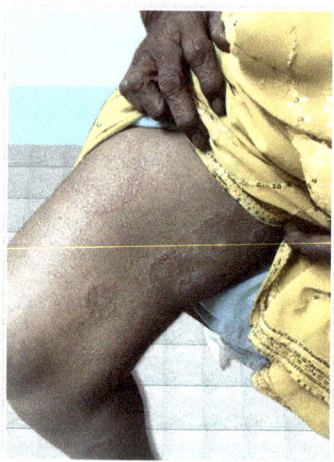

FIG. 9: Same patient as in figure 2.

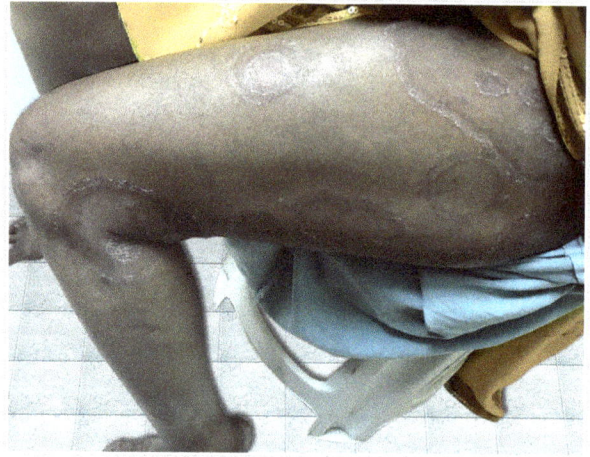

FIG. 10: Same patient as in figure 2.

Infections in Pregnancy

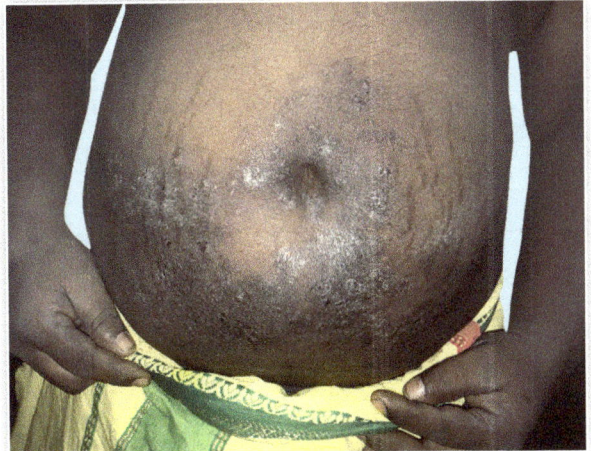

FIG. 11: Tinea corporis during second trimester in a diabetic patient.

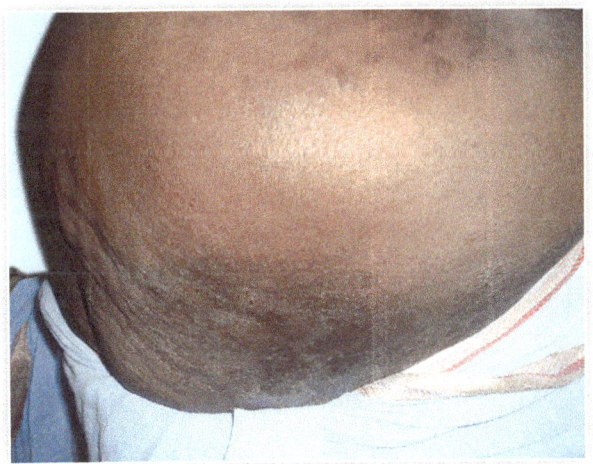

FIG. 12: Tinea involving waist area in a multipara.

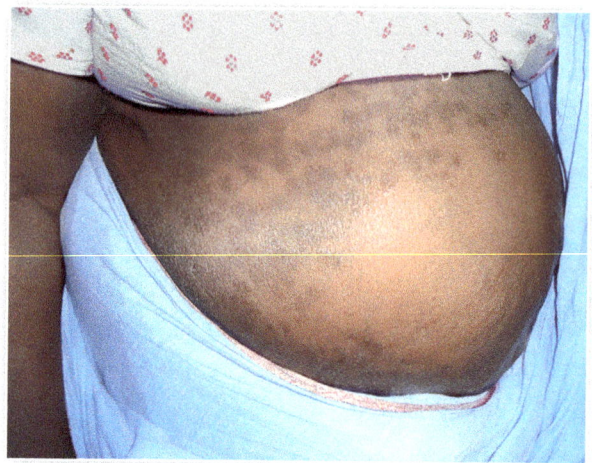

FIG. 13: Extensive tinea corporis in a pregnant woman.

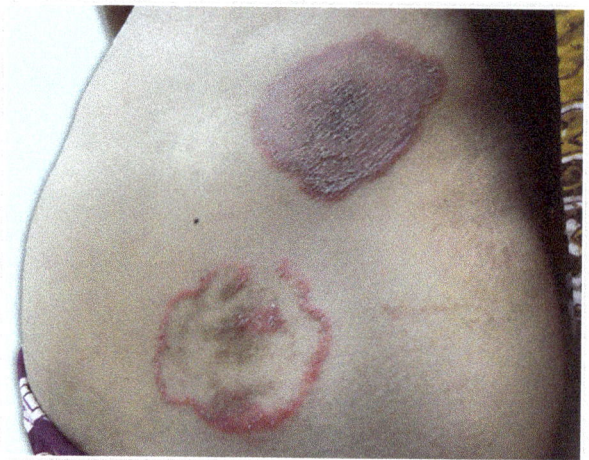

FIG. 14: Recurring infection in pregnancy.

Infections in Pregnancy

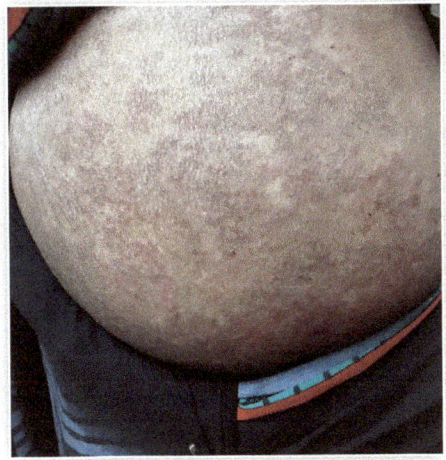

FIG. 15: Noninflammatory tinea corporis in a primi.

CHAPTER 12: Infections in Children

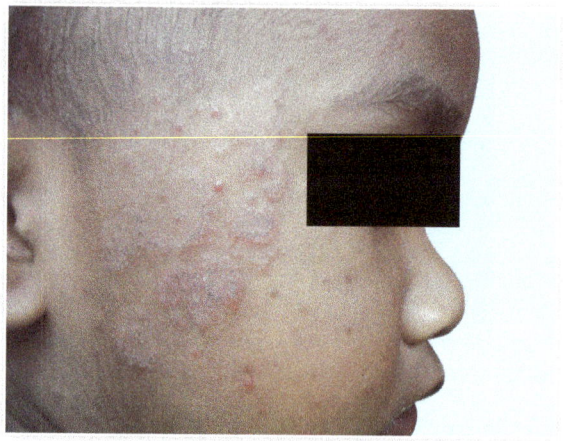

FIG. 1: Tinea faciei masquerading as atopic dermatitis.

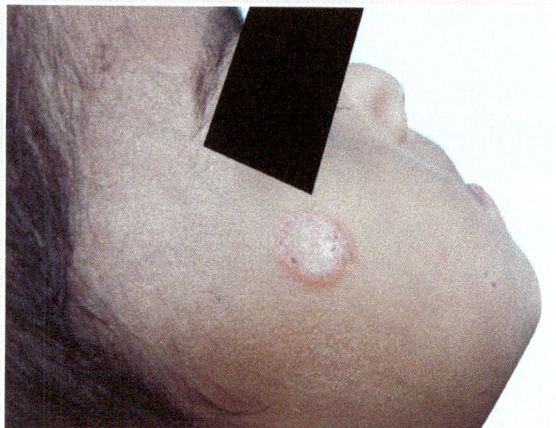

FIG. 2: Tinea faciei mimicking impetigo circinata.

Infections in Children

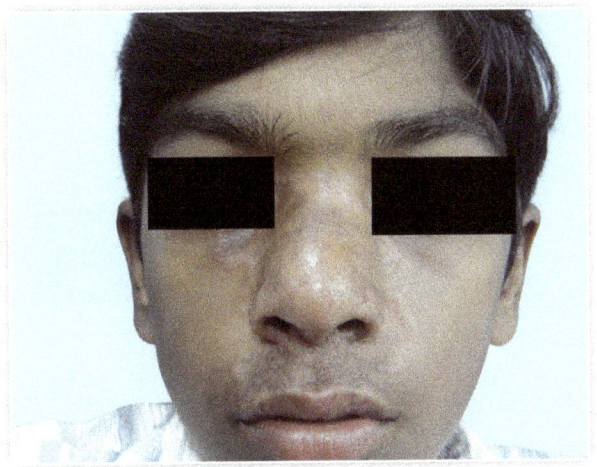

FIG. 3: Tinea faciei involving mucocutaneous junctions of eye, nose and mouth.

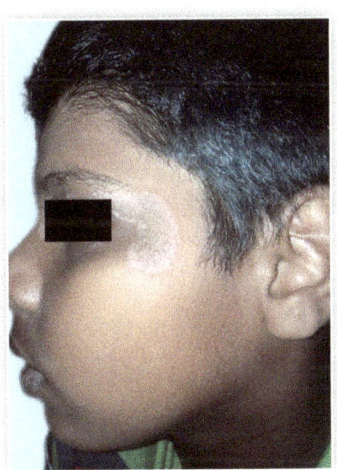

FIG. 4: Tinea faciei taking a linear morphology; responded to topical antifungal.

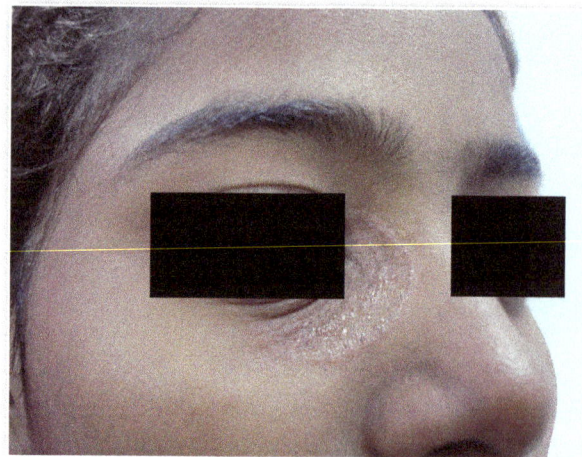

FIG. 5: Tinea faciei involving the chef tinea faciei eye.

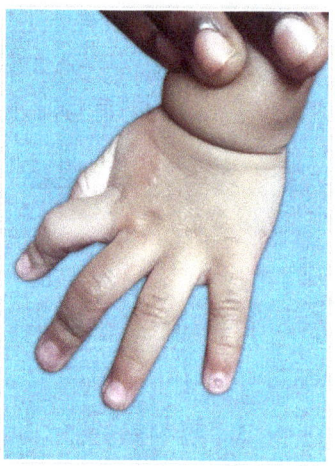

FIG. 6: Tinea manuum in an infant.

Infections in Children

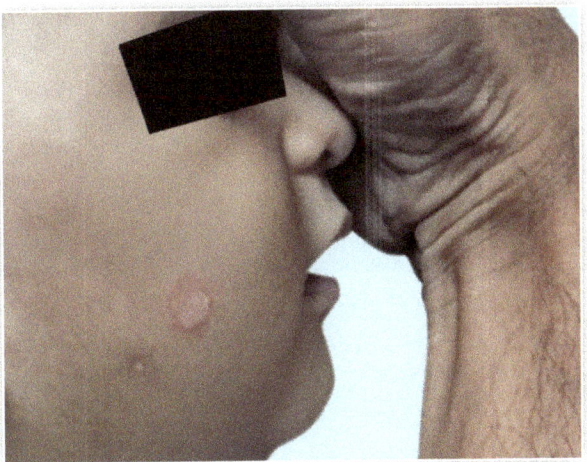

FIG. 7: Tinea faciei in an infant.

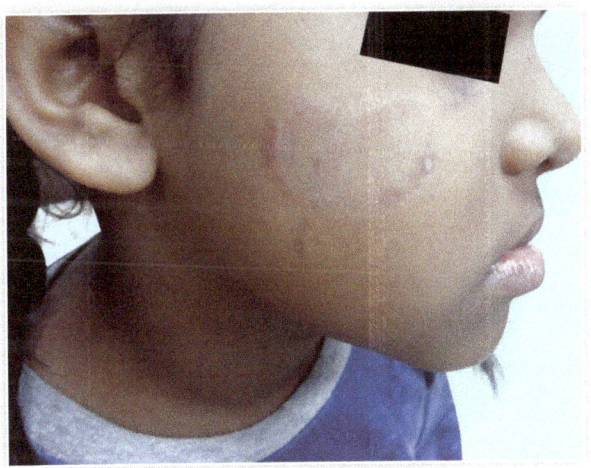

FIG. 8: Tinea faciei in a toddler.

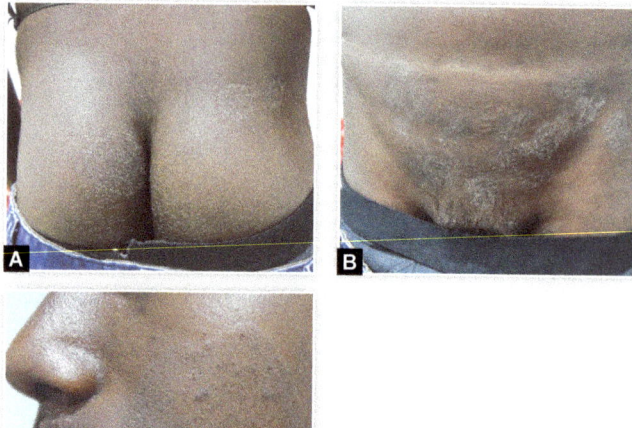

FIGS. 9A TO C: Disseminated dermatophytosis in a hosteller.

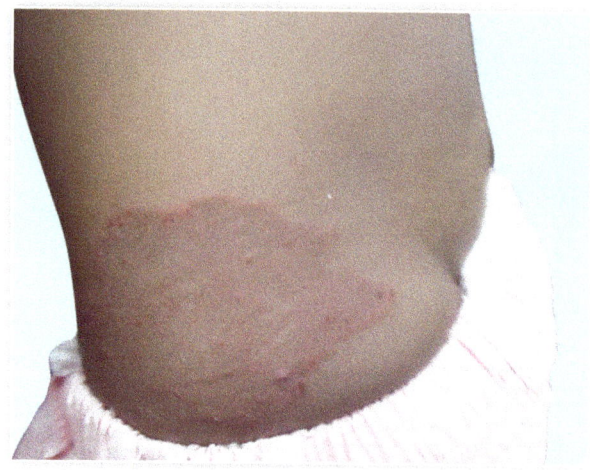

FIG. 10: Waist involvement tight occlusive dress may contribute.

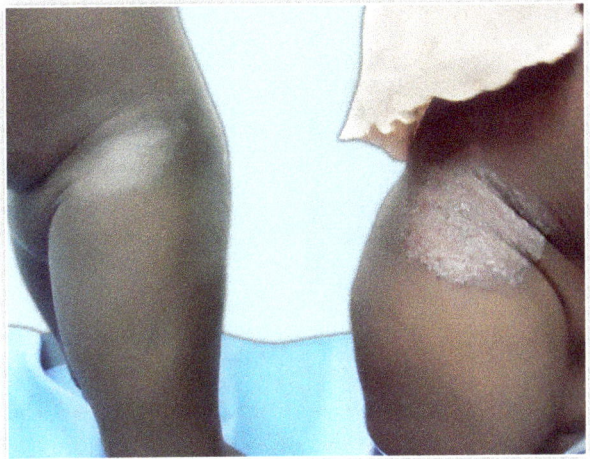

FIG. 11: Tinea corporis in twins.

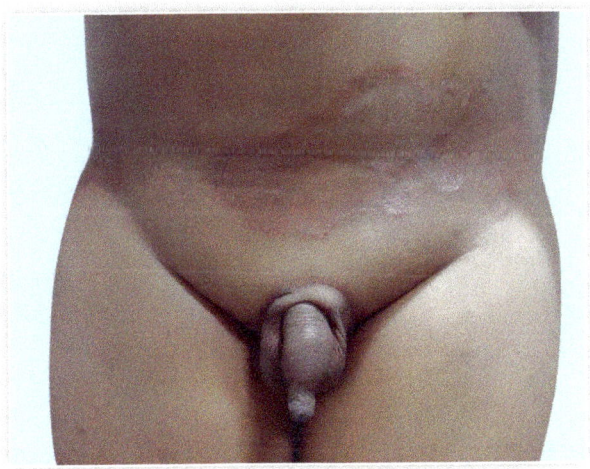

FIG. 12: Waist involvement in a child contacted from mother.

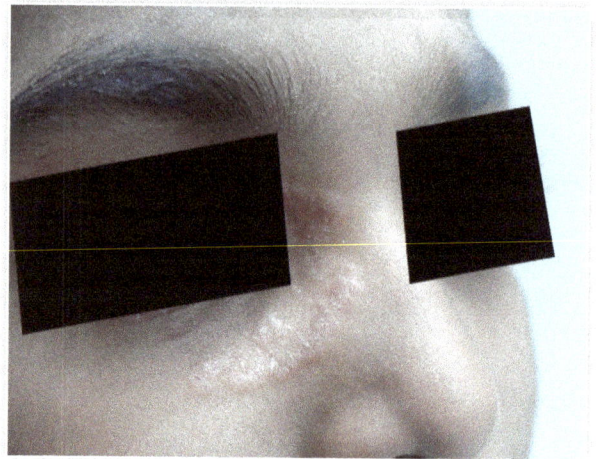

FIG. 13: Tinea faciei in a child.

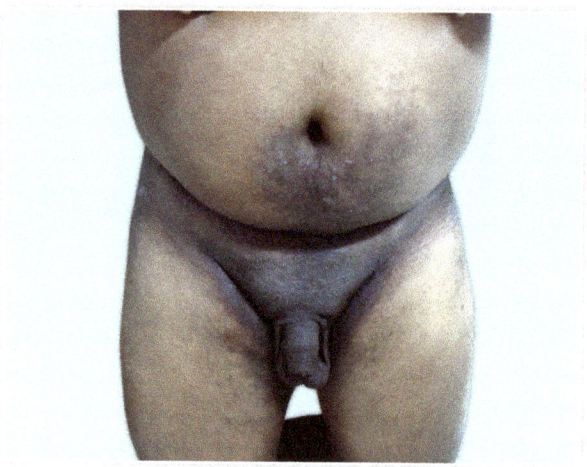

FIG. 14: Pigmentation following treatment in a child.

Infections in Children

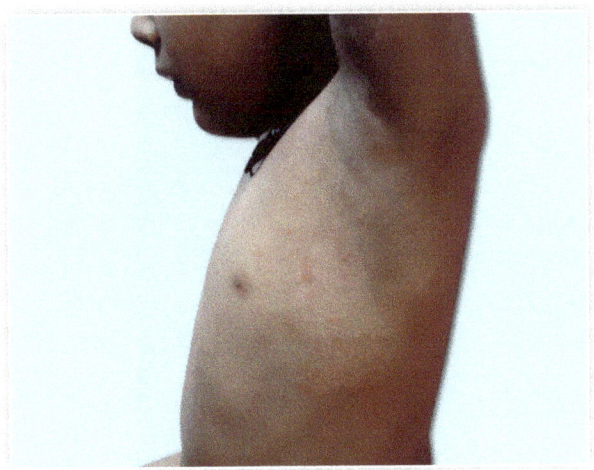

FIG. 15: Extensive involvement of the axilla.

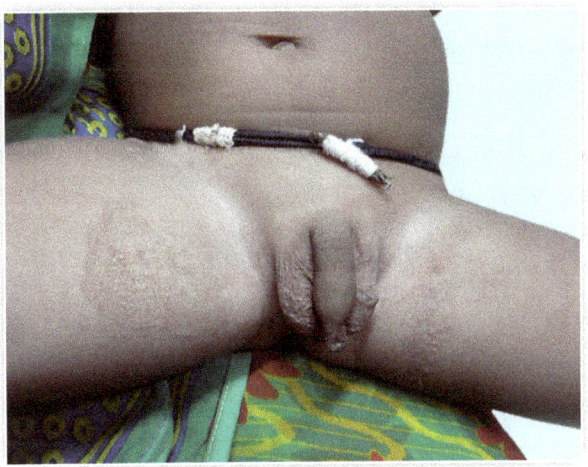

FIG. 16: Extensive tinea cruris.

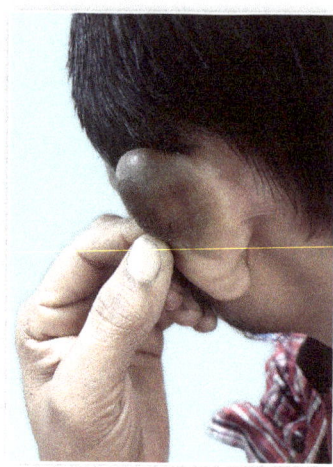

FIG. 17: Tinea infection behind the left ear.

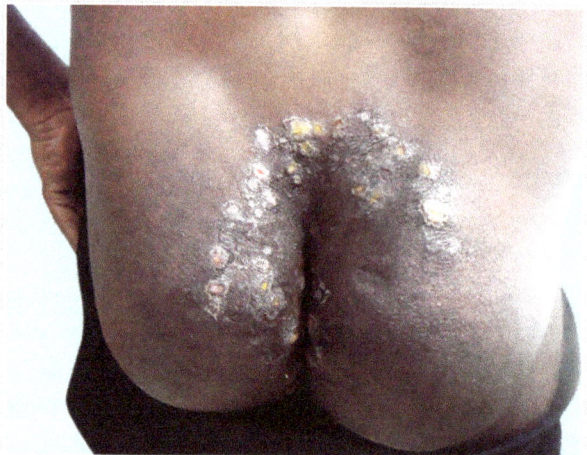

FIG. 18: Impetiginization following treatment of tinea glutealis.

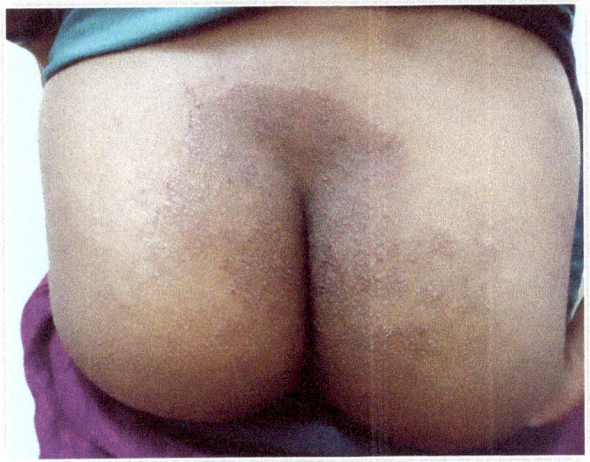

FIG. 19: Postinflammatory pigmentation following treatment.

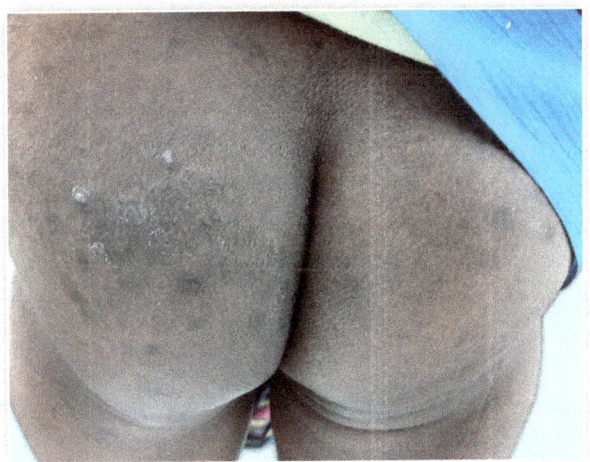

FIG. 20: Gluteal involvement in a child.

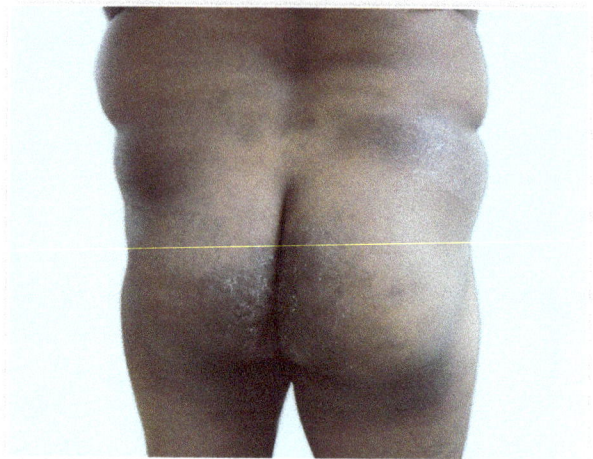

FIG. 21: Tinea glutealis and corporis in a child.

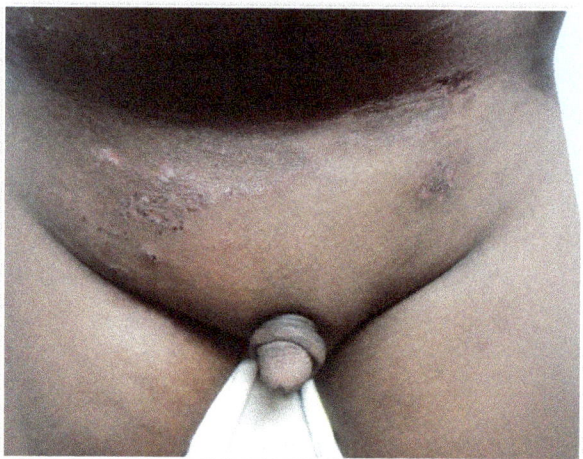

FIG. 22: Tinea corporis in an infant.

Infections in Children

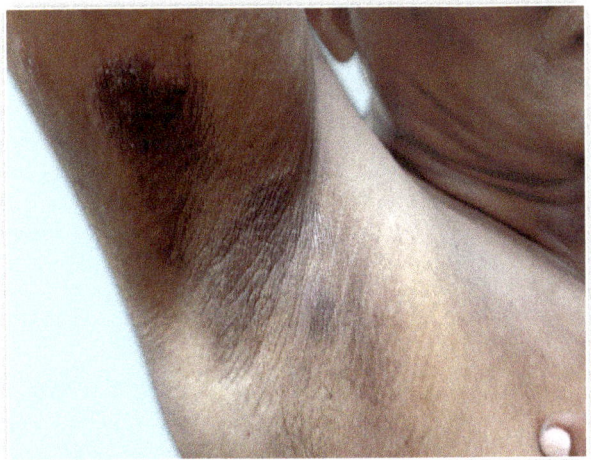

FIG. 23: Tinea axillaris in a child.

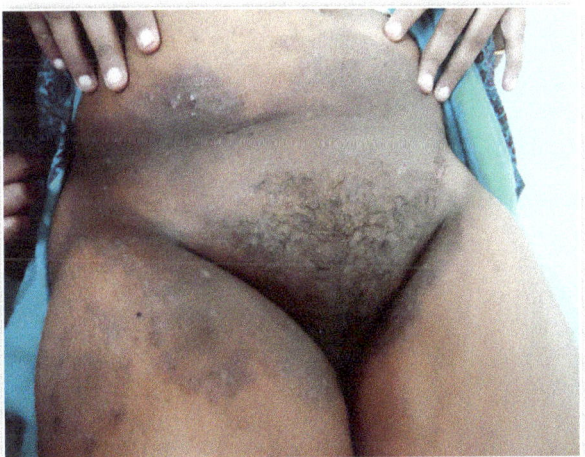

FIG. 24: Extensive involvement of the genital area and lower abdomen.

Color Atlas of Dermatophytoses: *Focus on Superficial Fungal Infections*

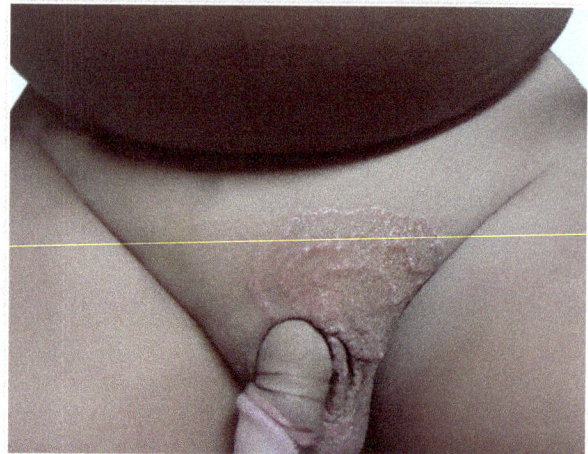

FIG. 25: Ring within ring appearance in a child.

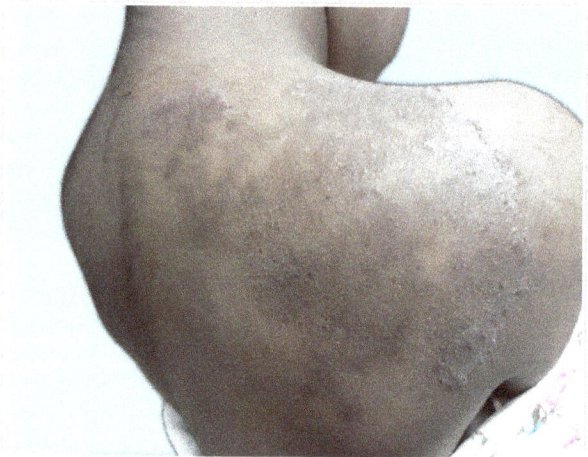

FIG. 26: Extensive tinea corporis in a child.

Infections in Children

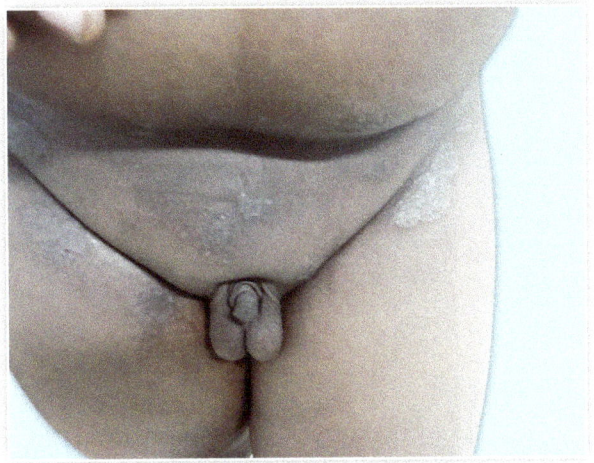

FIG. 27: Tinea corporis and cruris.

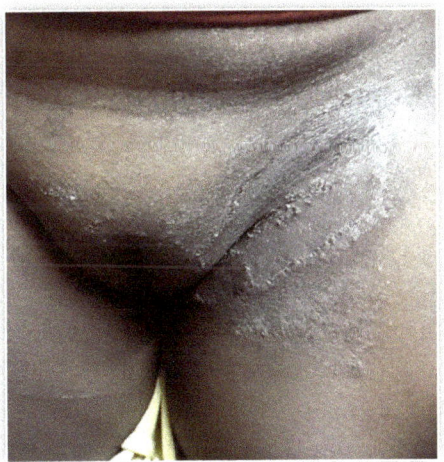

FIG. 28: Tinea cruris involving one side.

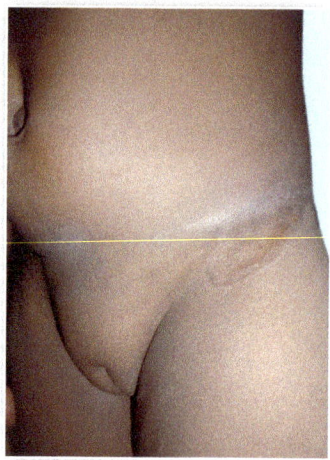

FIG. 29: Mimicking herald patch of pityriasis rosea.

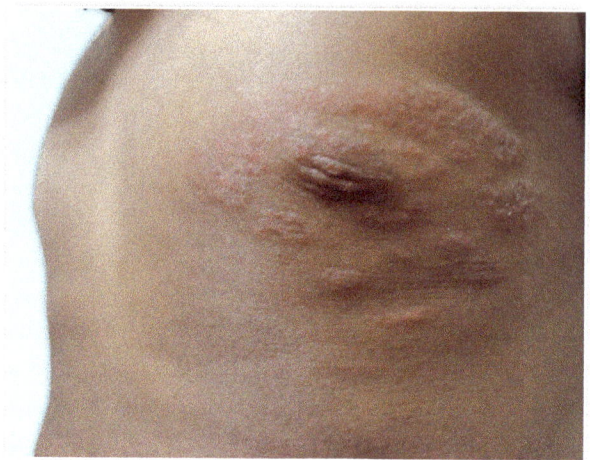

FIG. 30: Rare involvement of periareolar area.

Infections in Children

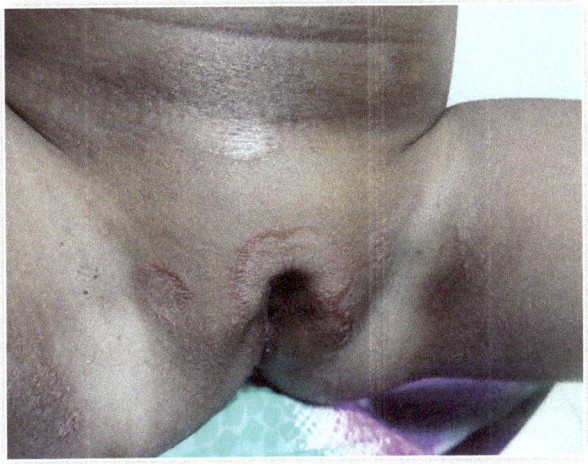

FIG. 31: Dermatophyte affecting the genital area groin and lower abdomen.

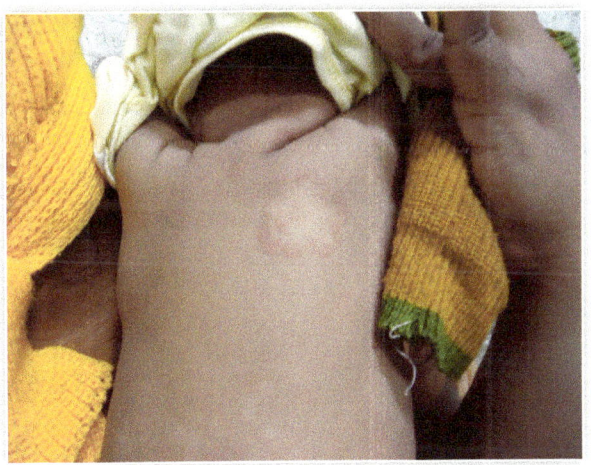

FIG. 32: Multiple patches of dermatophytosis.

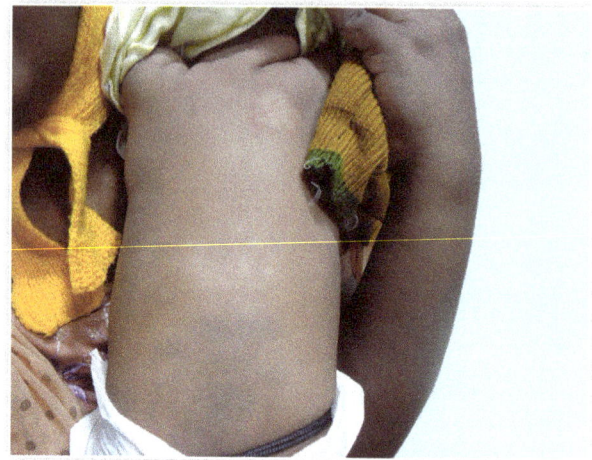

FIG. 33: Same patient as in figure 32. Note the well-defined margin.

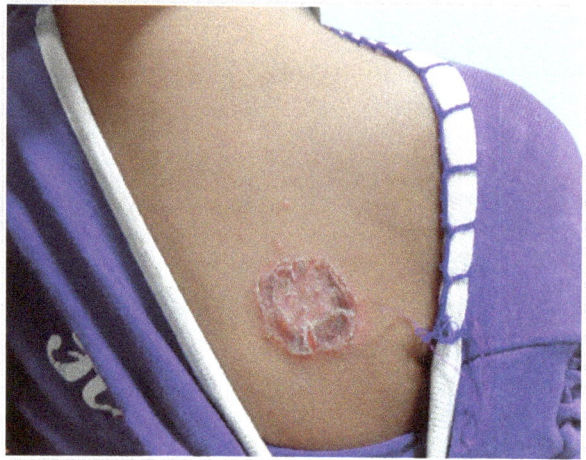

FIG. 34: Inflammatory type in a child.

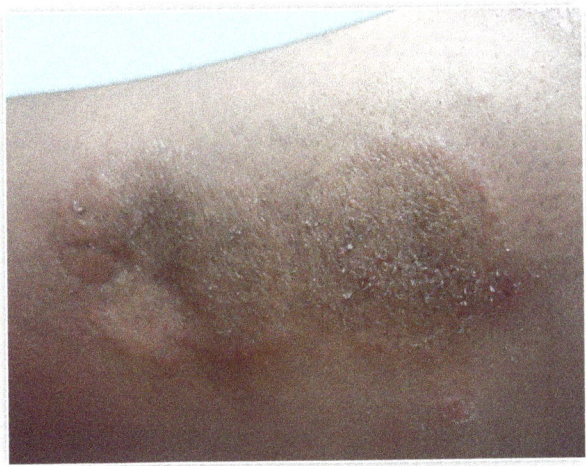

FIG. 35: Extensive limb involvement in a child.

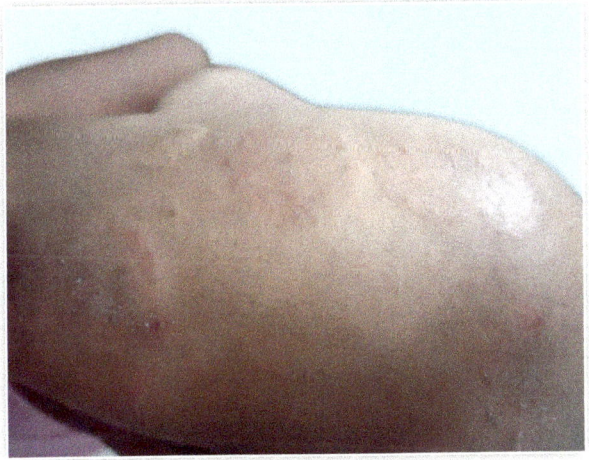

FIG. 36: Truncal involvement in a child.

Color Atlas of Dermatophytoses: *Focus on Superficial Fungal Infections*

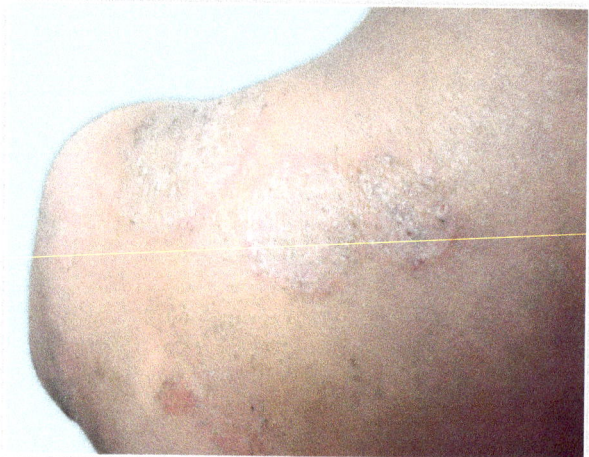

FIG. 37: Back involvement in a child.

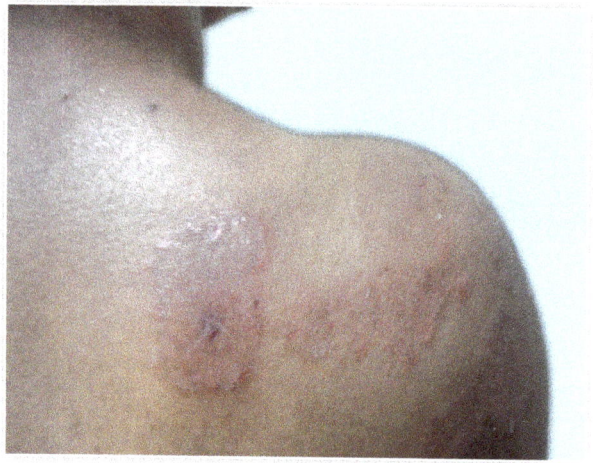

FIG. 38: Same patient as in figure 37.

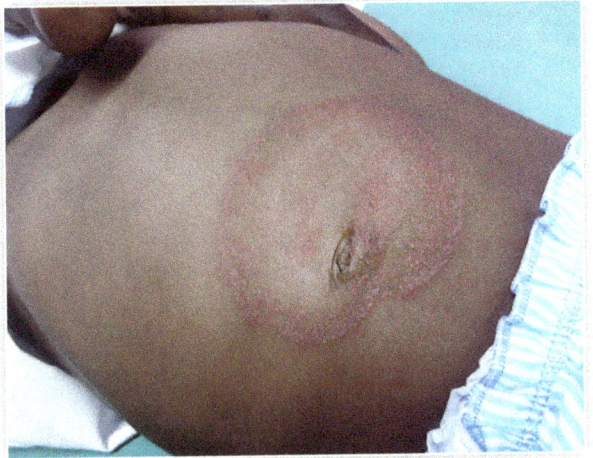

FIG. 39: Classical annular patch with well-defined margin.

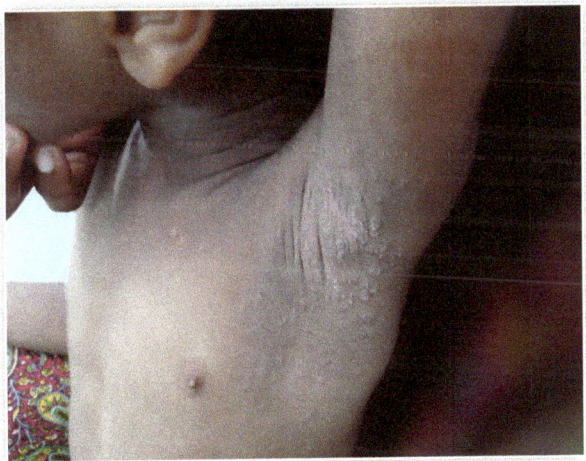

FIG. 40: Tinea axillaris in a child.

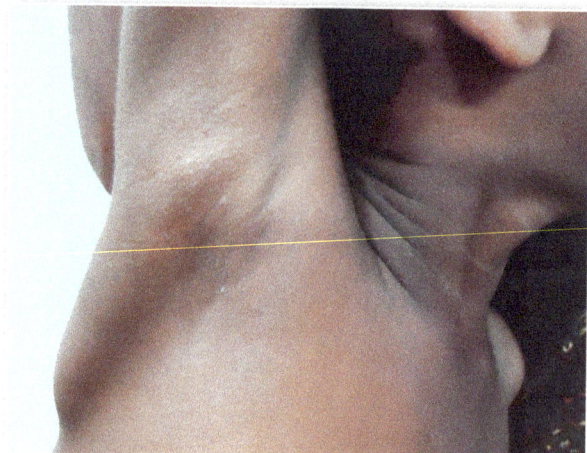

FIG. 41: Same patient as in figure 40.

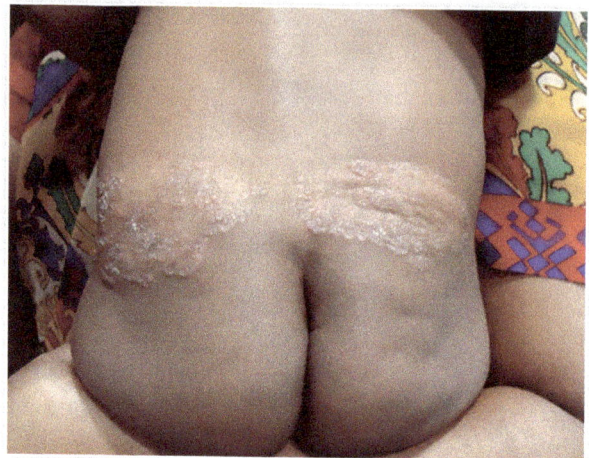

FIG. 42: Extensive waist involvement.

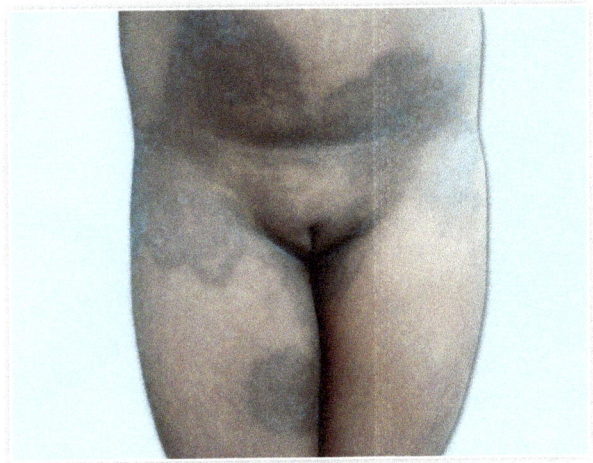

FIG. 43: Post-treatment pigmentation.

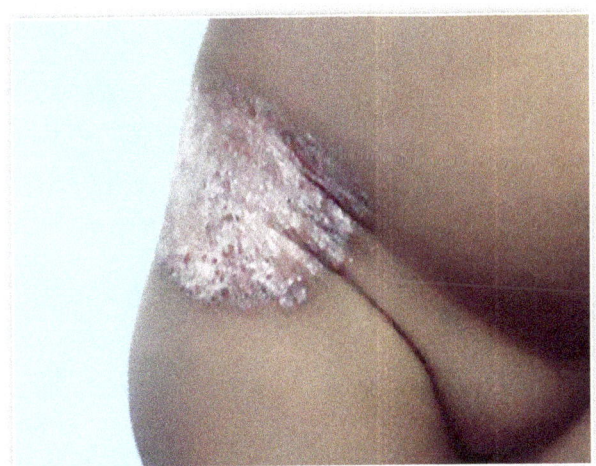

FIG. 44: Waist involvement in a child.

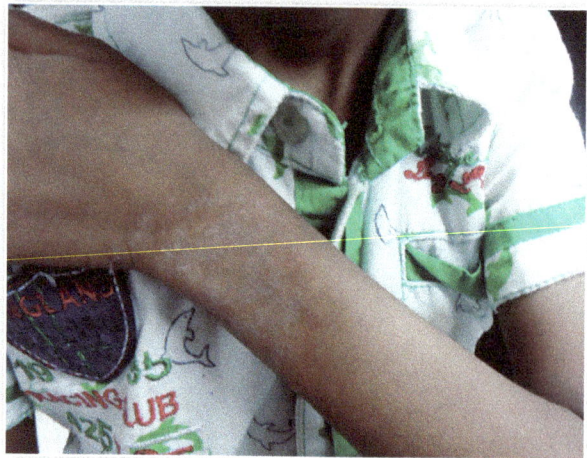

FIG. 45: Involvement of wrist in a child.

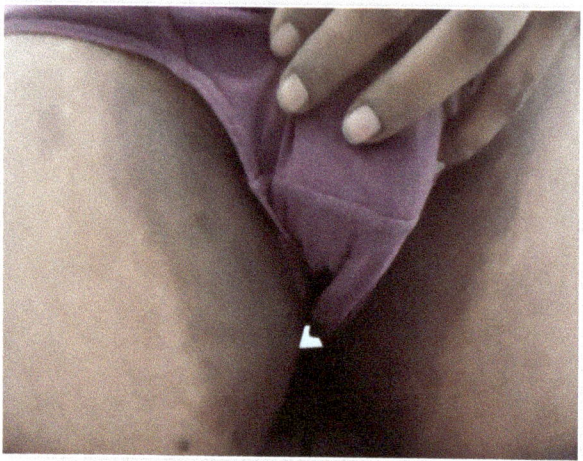

FIG. 46: Tinea cruris in a child.

Infections in Children

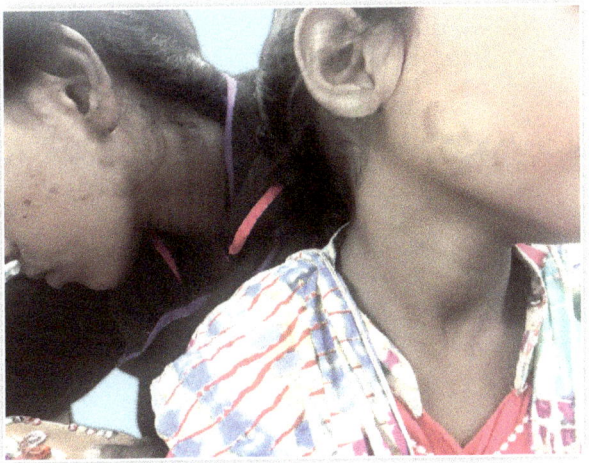

FIG. 47: Tinea faciei in sisters.

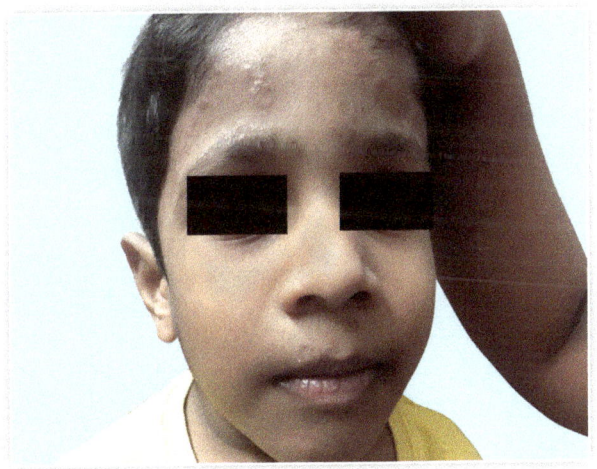

FIG. 48: Multiple small patches of tinea faciei in a child.

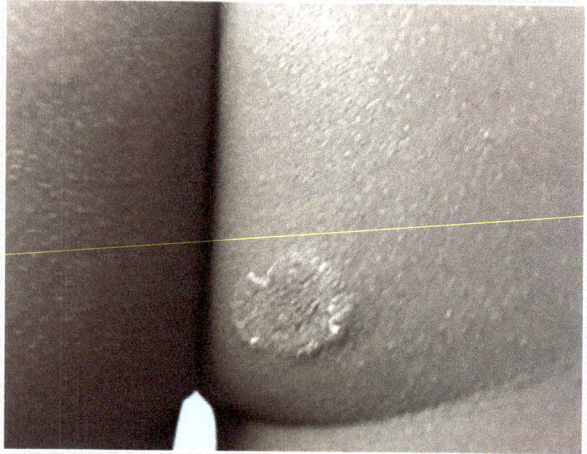

FIG. 49: Tinea faciei in a child mother having tinea manuum.

CHAPTER 13: Infections in Adolescent

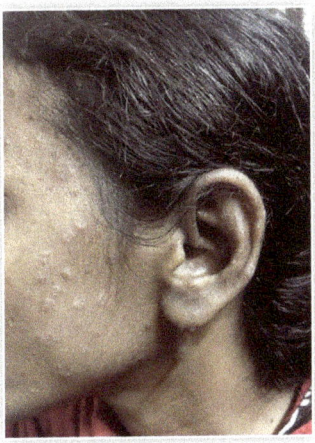

FIG. 1: Teenage girl with scaly patch over the face and ear.

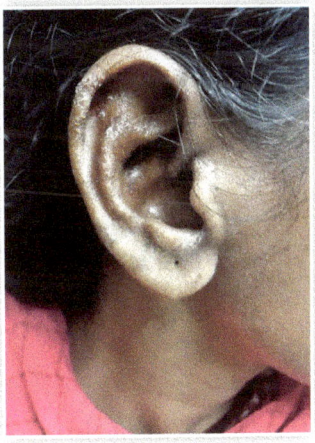

FIG. 2: Involvement of right pinna as well.

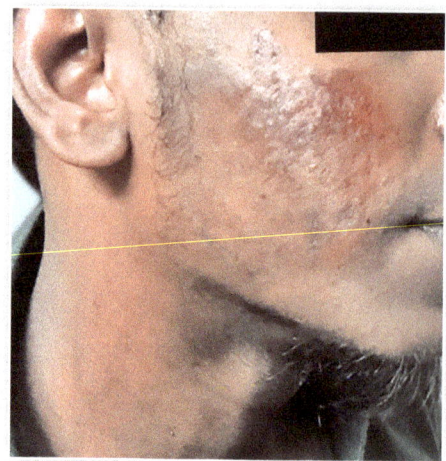

FIG. 3: Tinea faciei in an adolescent.

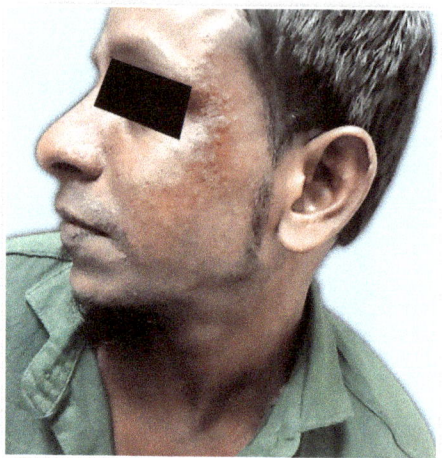

FIG. 4: Same patient as in figure 3, note bilateral involvement.

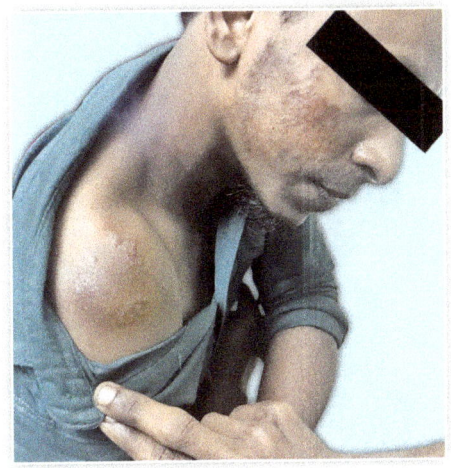

FIG. 5: Tinea corporis in same patient as in figures 3 and 4.

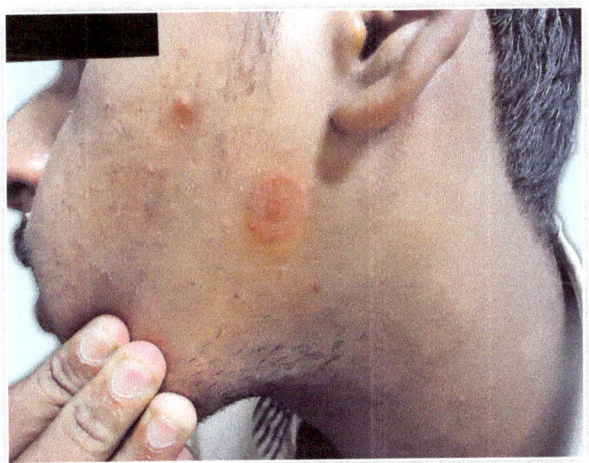

FIG. 6: Tinea faciei in an adolescent having acne.

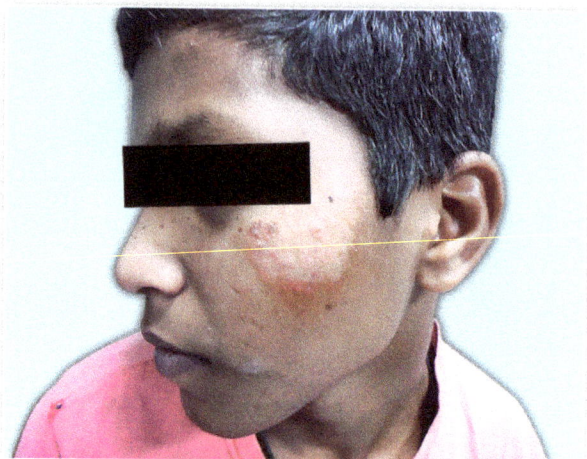

FIG. 7: Tinea faciei, margin well-defined below and ill-defined above.

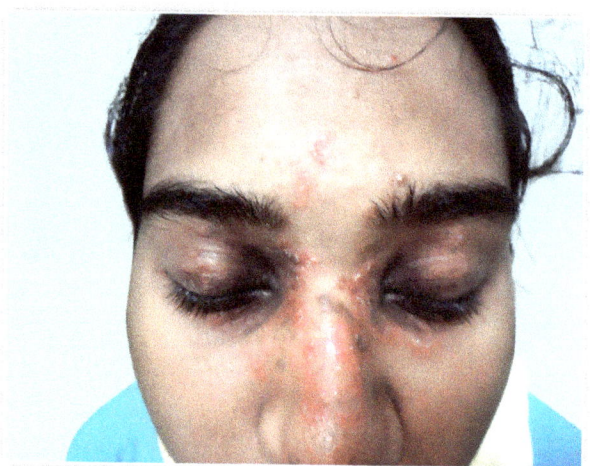

FIG. 8: Inflammatory tinea involving the central face.

Infections in Adolescent

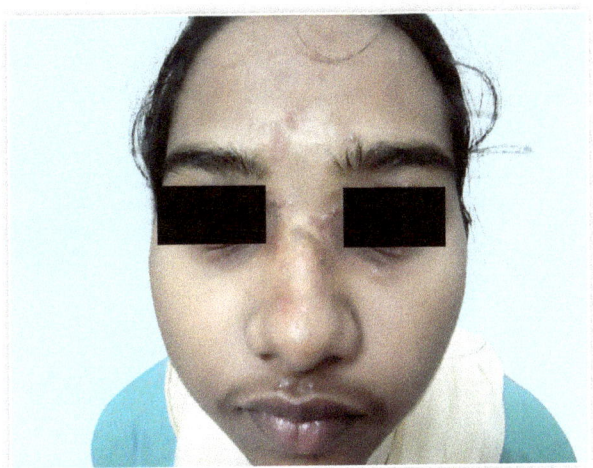

FIG. 9: Same patient as in figure 8 after one week of treatment.

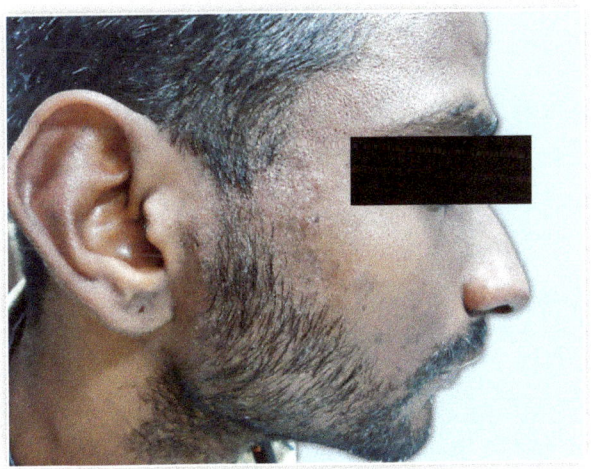

FIG. 10: Tinea barbae in a youth which can be easily missed.

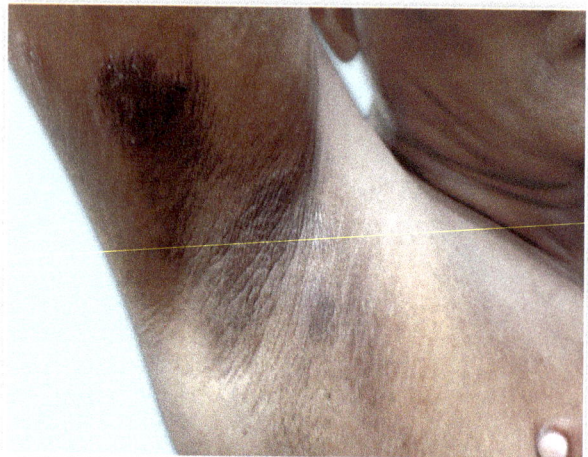

FIG. 11: Tinea axillaris in a college student.

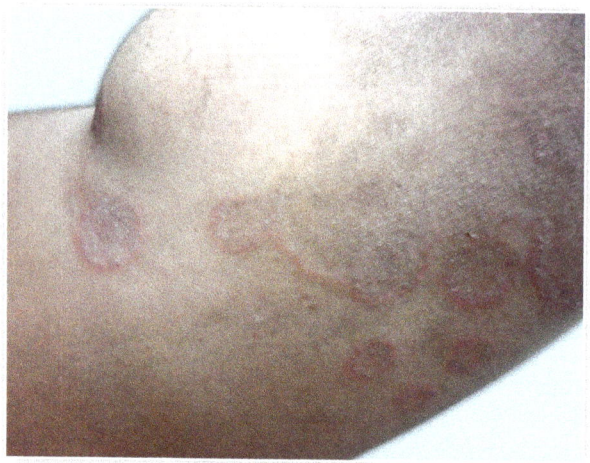

FIG. 12: Patches involving the upper arm.

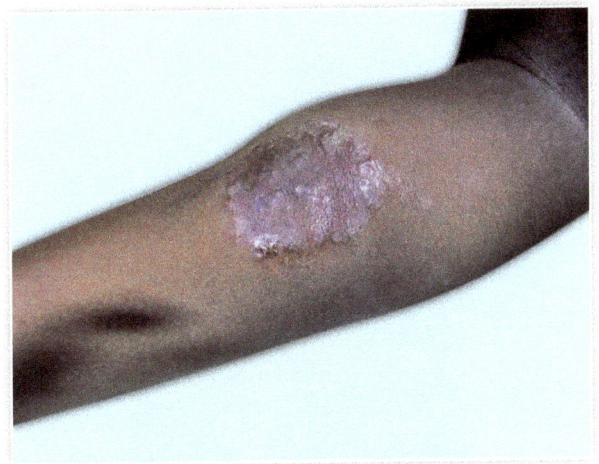

FIG. 13: Tinea corporis without central clearance mimicking eczema.

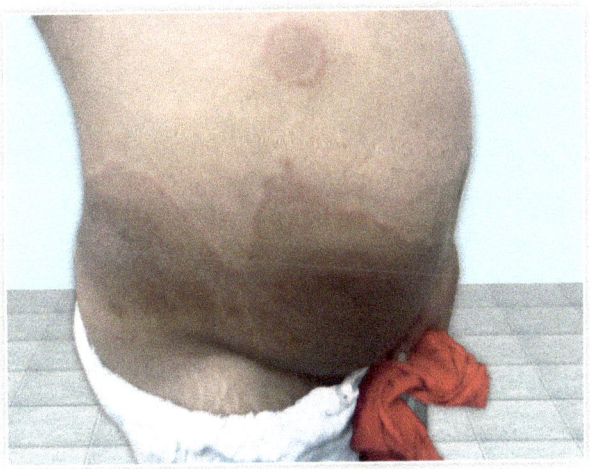

FIG. 14: Adolescent with tinea corporis around the waist and the abdomen.

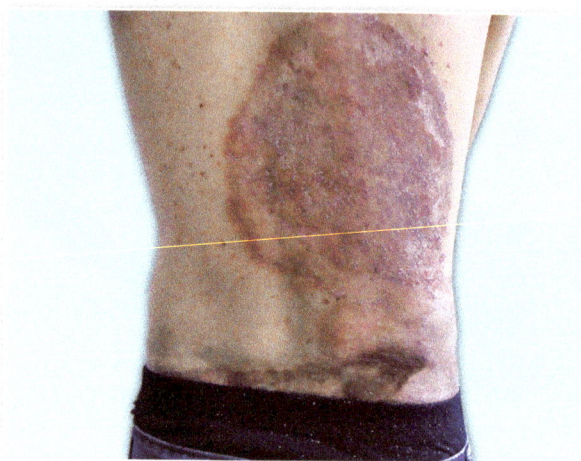

FIG. 15: Extensive involvement teenager same as in figure 14.

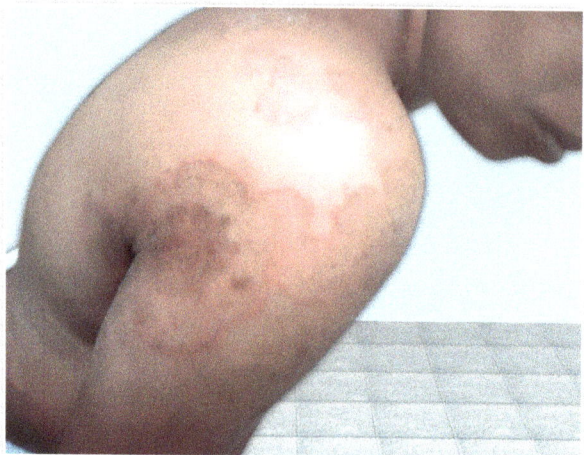

FIG. 16: Coalescing patches of tinea corporis showing clearance in some places.

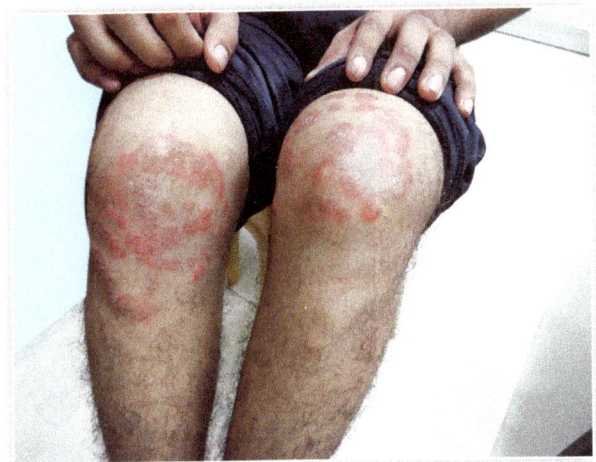

FIG. 17: Bilateral involvement of the knees mimicking psoriasis.

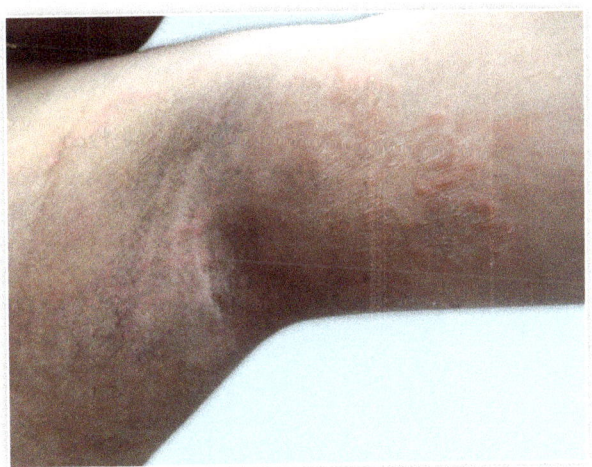

FIG. 18: Extensive dermatophytoses.

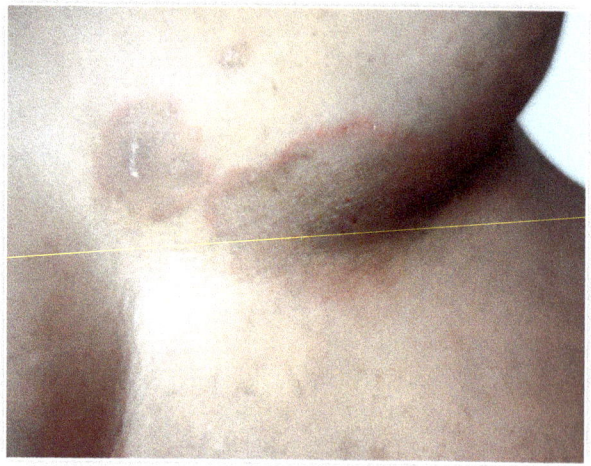

FIG. 19: Extensive dermatophytoses, same patient as in figure 18.

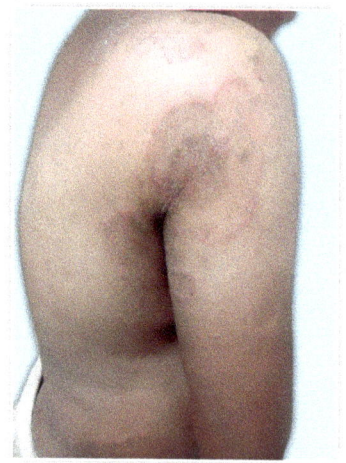

FIG. 20: Extensive dermatophytoses, same patient as in figure 19.

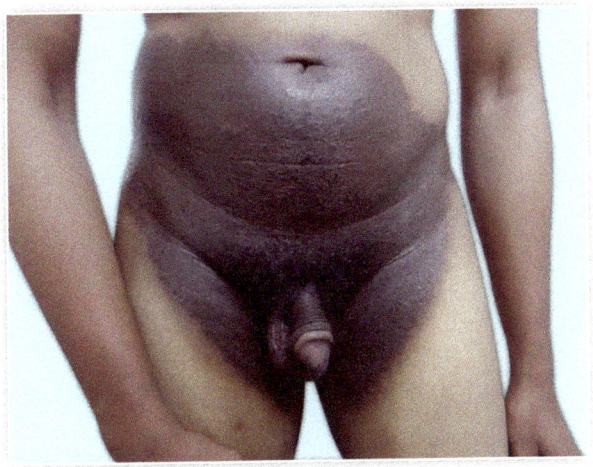

FIG. 21: Pigmentation post-treatment in widespread tinea corporis.

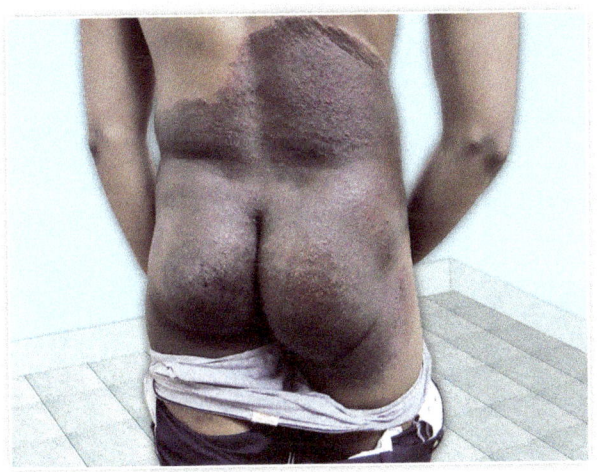

FIG. 22: Same patient as in figure 21.

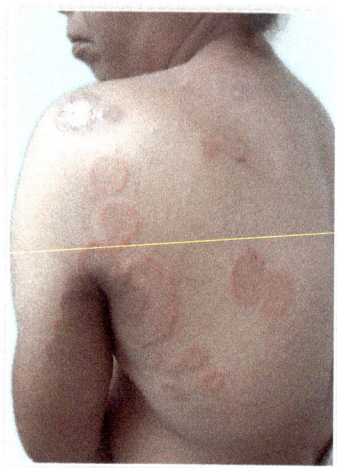

FIG. 23: Scaly extensive lesion recalcitrant to treatment.

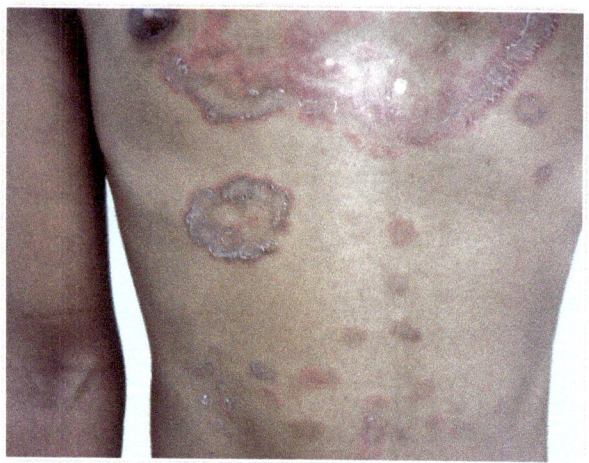

FIG. 24: Tinea imbricata.

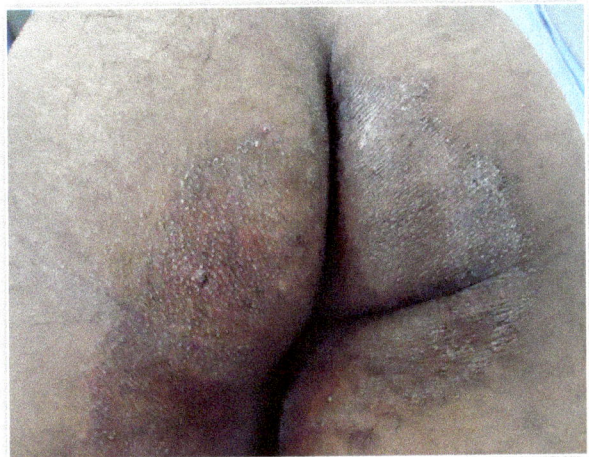

FIG. 25: Tinea glutealis with follicular keratosis.

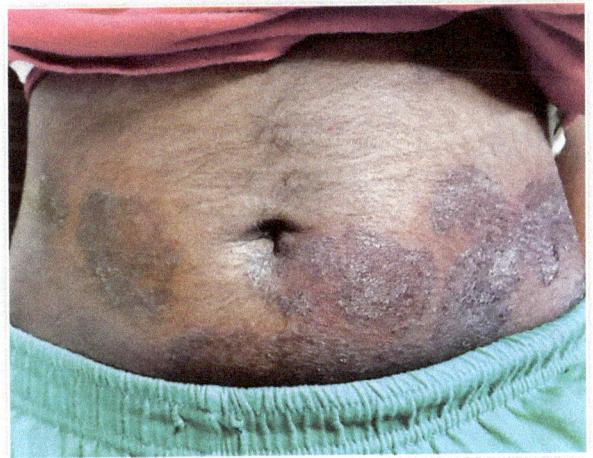

FIG. 26: Dobi itch in a teenager.

Color Atlas of Dermatophytoses: *Focus on Superficial Fungal Infections*

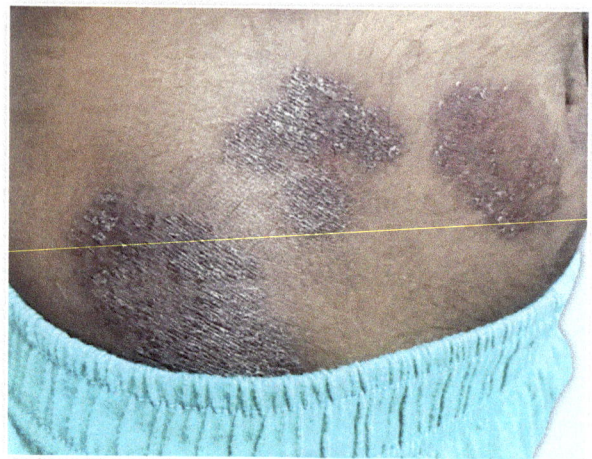

FIG. 27: Same patient as in figure 26.

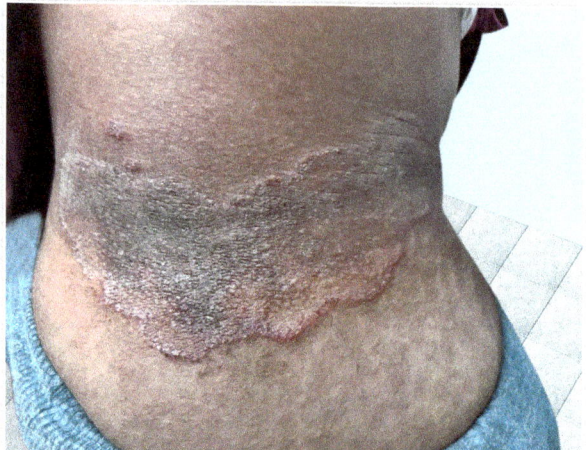

FIG. 28: Classical waist involvement in an adolescent.

Infections in Adolescent

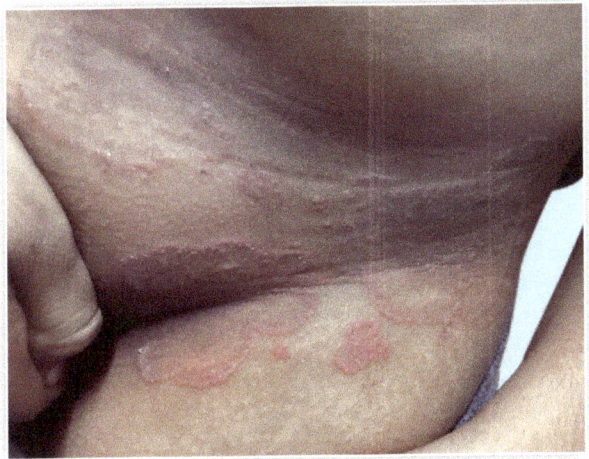

FIG. 29: Same patient as in figure 28 showing involvement of groin and genitals.

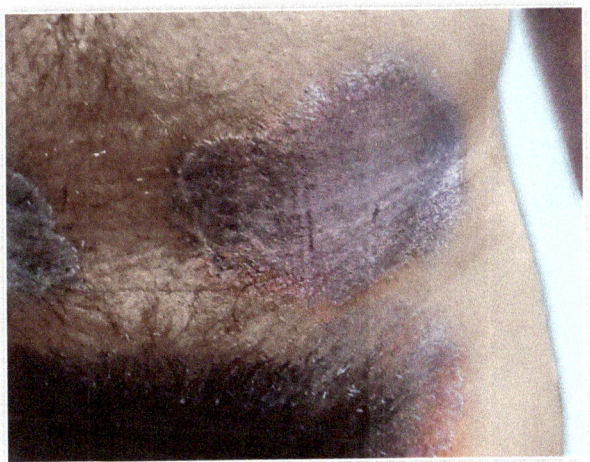

FIG. 30: Asymptomatic patches of tinea corporis and cruris.

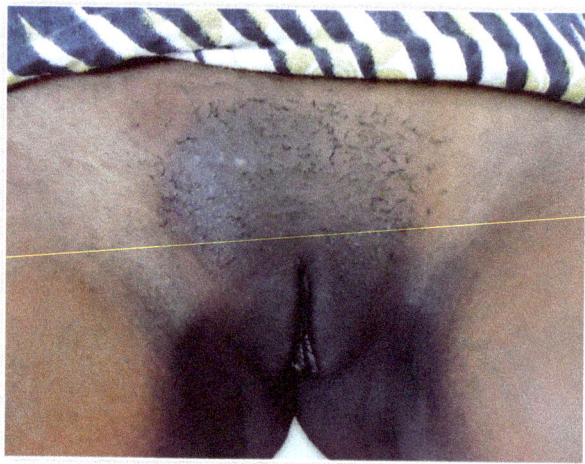

FIG. 31: Pigmentation following treatment for dermatophytosis.

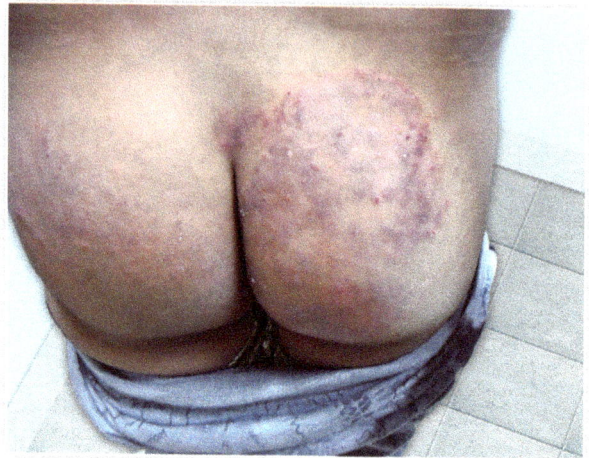

FIG. 32: Tinea glutealis unilateral involvement in an adolescent.

Infections in Adolescent

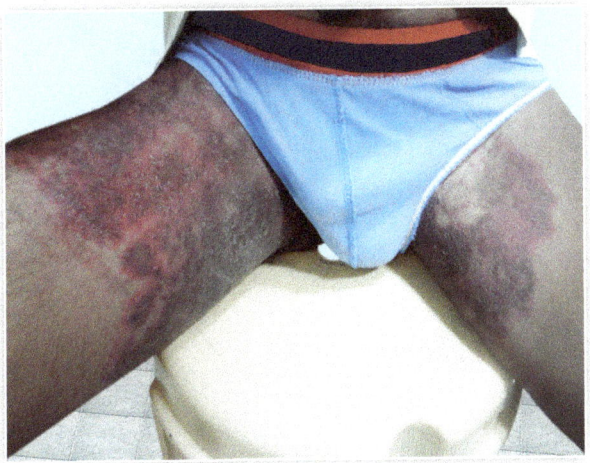

FIG. 33: Extensive tinea cruris.

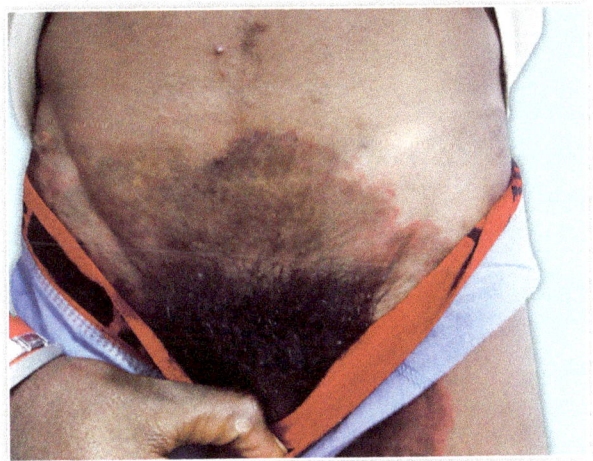

FIG. 34: Same patient as in figure 33.

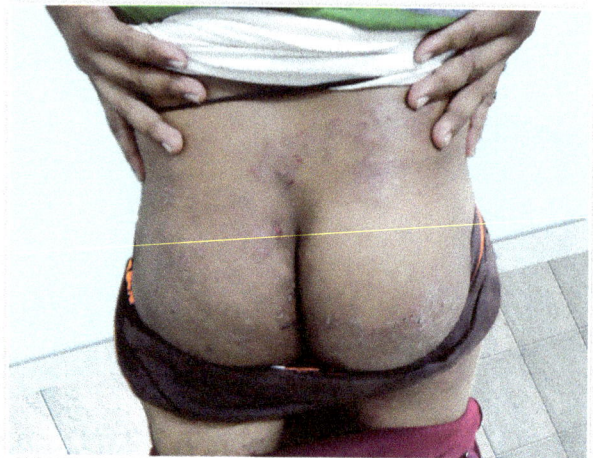

FIG. 35: Note bilateral involvement in a teenager.

CHAPTER 14: Infections in the Immunocompromised

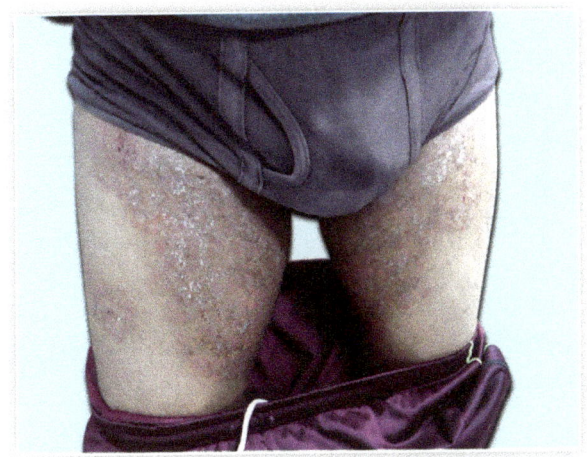

FIG. 1: Extensive tinea cruris in a man on immunosuppressive therapy.

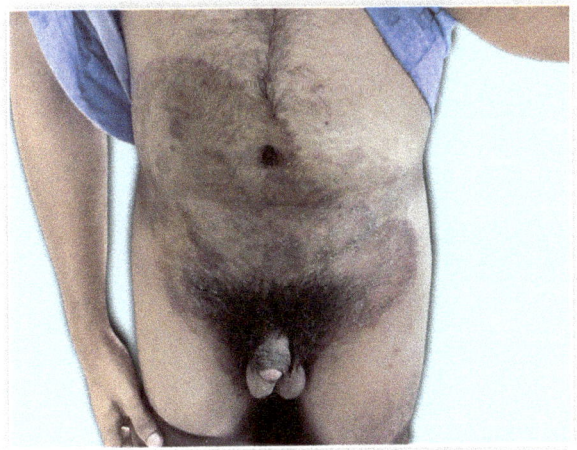

FIG. 2: Extensive involvement in a patient on antituberculosis drugs.

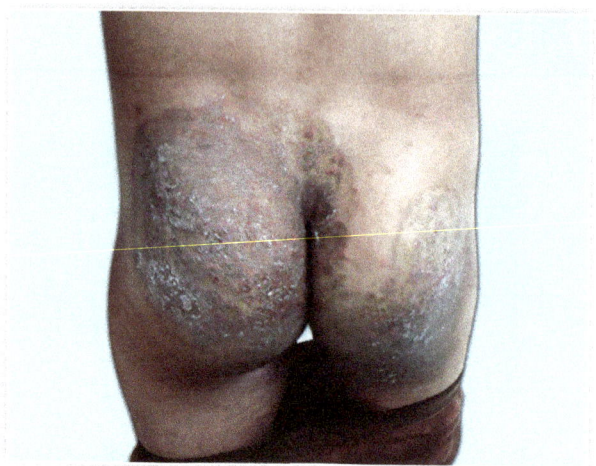

FIG. 3: Same patient as in figure 2.

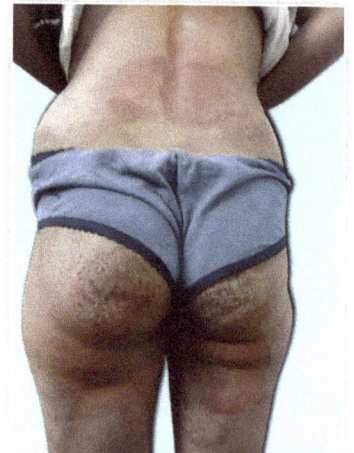

FIG. 4: Patient on systemic steroid.

Infections in the Immunocompromised

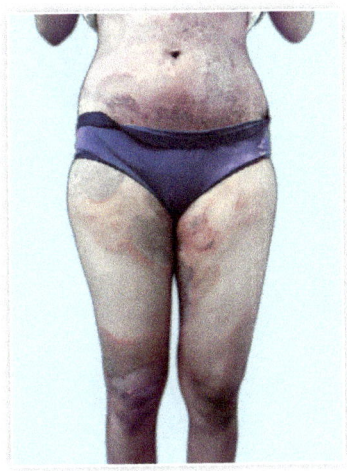

FIG. 5: Same patient as in figure 4.

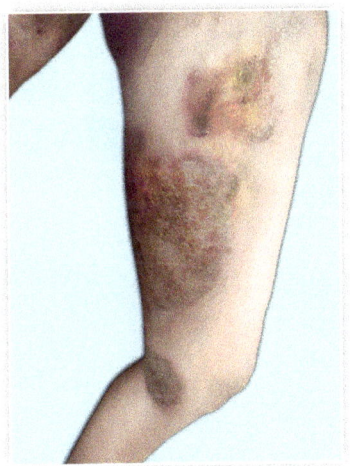

FIG. 6: Same patient as in figure 4.

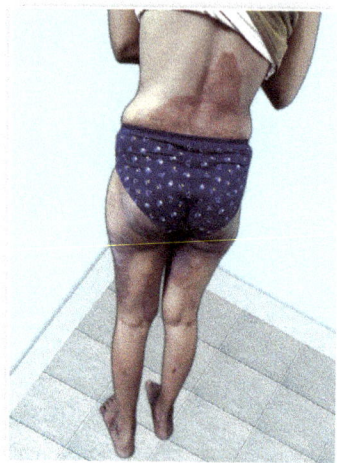

FIG. 7: Same patient as in figure 4 after treatment.

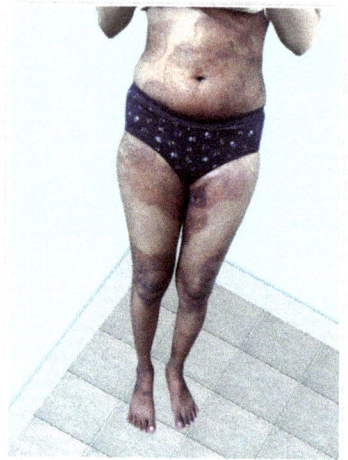

FIG. 8: Same patient as in figure 4.

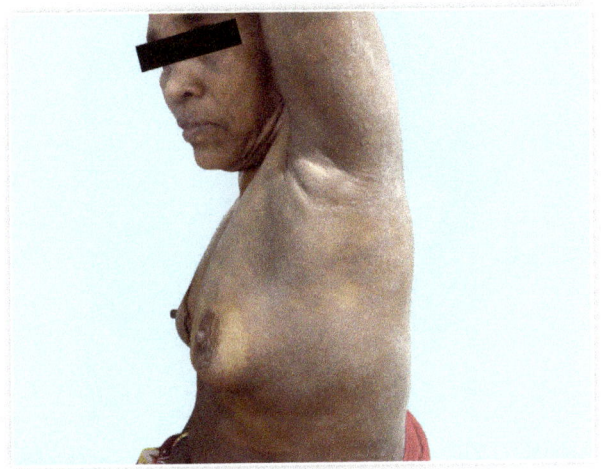

FIG. 9: Extensive dermatophyte detected to have diabetes.

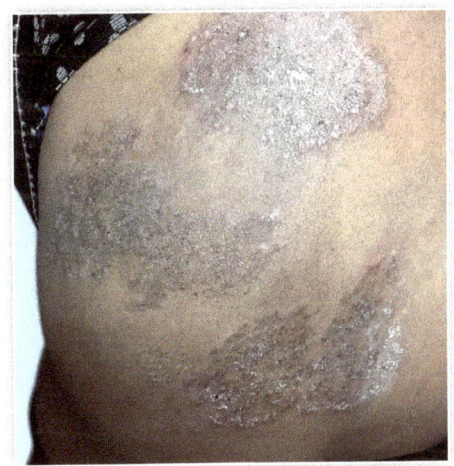

FIG. 10: Extensive dermatophytosis in a lady with uncontrolled diabetes.

Color Atlas of Dermatophytoses: *Focus on Superficial Fungal Infections*

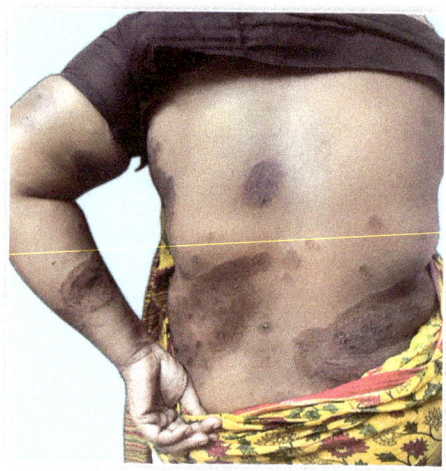

FIG. 11: Extensive tinea corporis in a patient on cyclosporine.

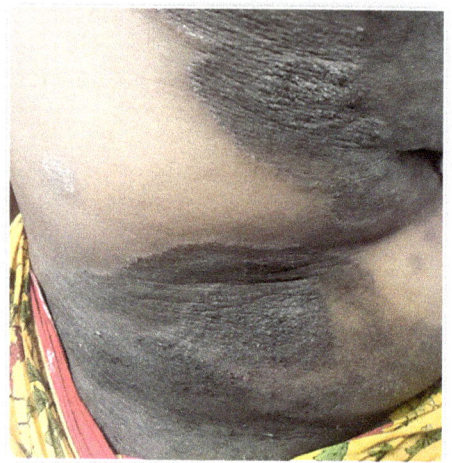

FIG. 12: Same patient as in figure 11.

Infections in the Immunocompromised

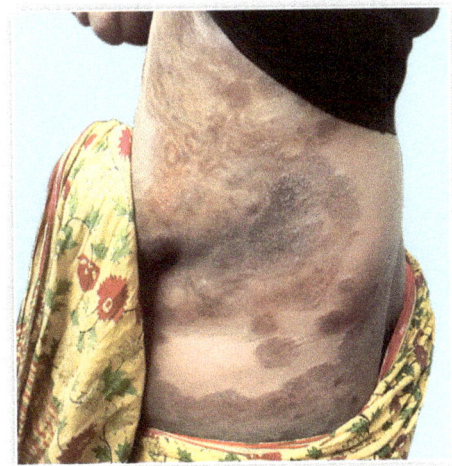

FIG. 13: Same patient as in figure 11.

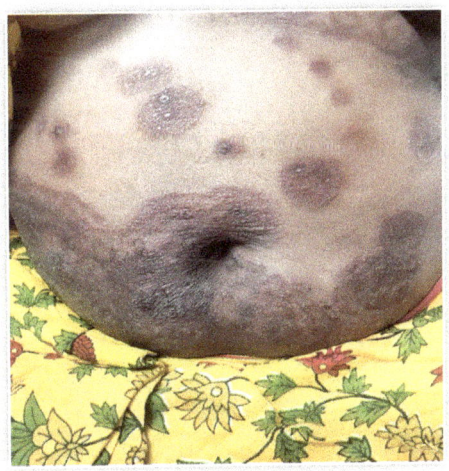

FIG. 14: Same patient as in figure 11.

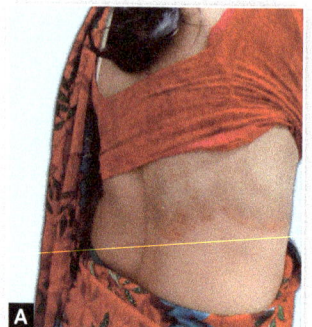 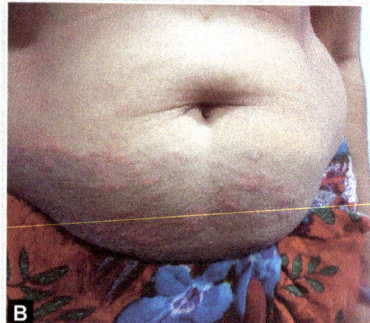

FIGS. 15A AND B: Tinea corporis in a diabetic patient.

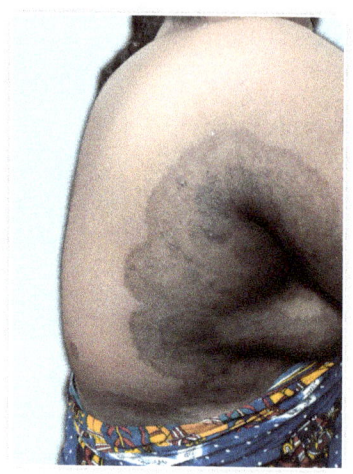

FIG. 16: Same patient as in figure 12 after treatment.

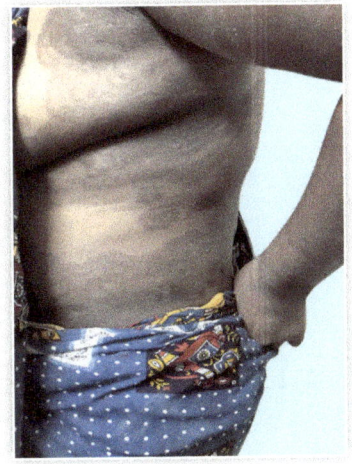

FIG. 17: Same patient as in figure 13 after treatment.

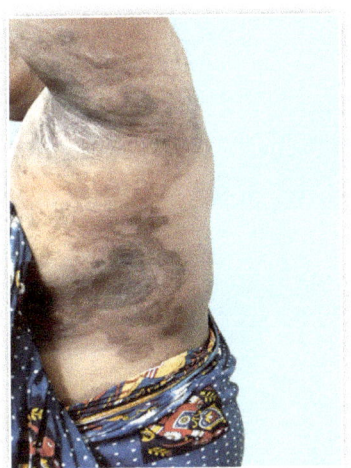

FIG. 18: Same patient as in figure 13 after treatment.

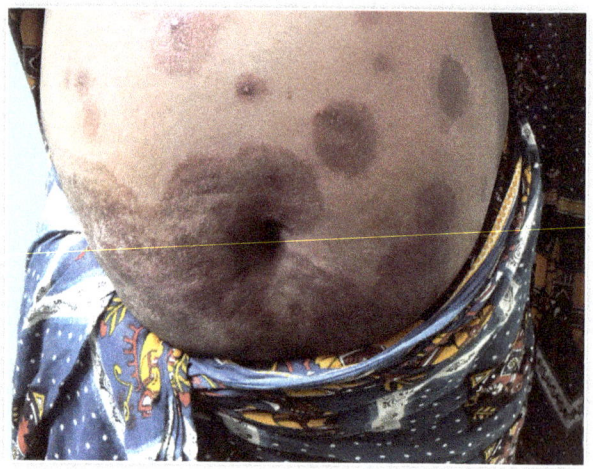

FIG. 19: Same patient as in figure 14.

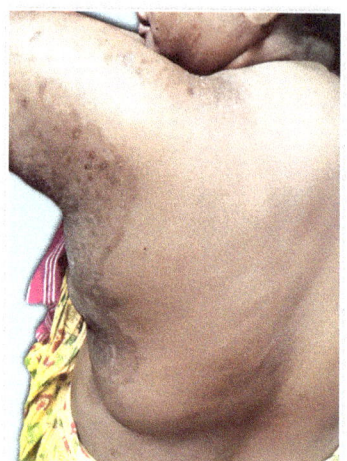

FIG. 20: Same patient as in figure 15.

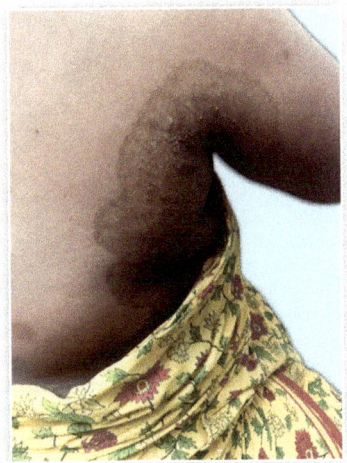

FIG. 21: Same patient as in figure 16.

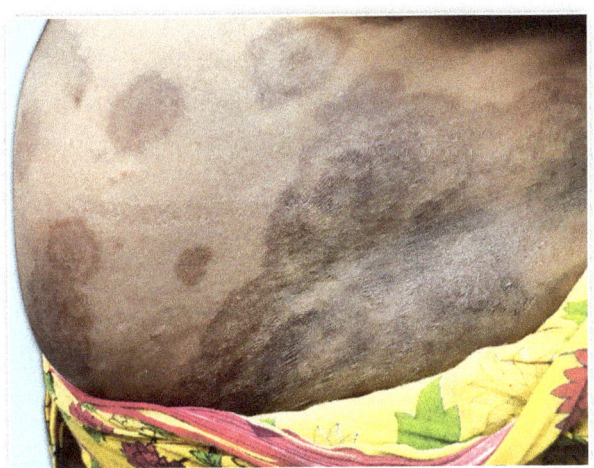

FIG. 22: Same patient as in figure 17 scraping negative after complete treatment.

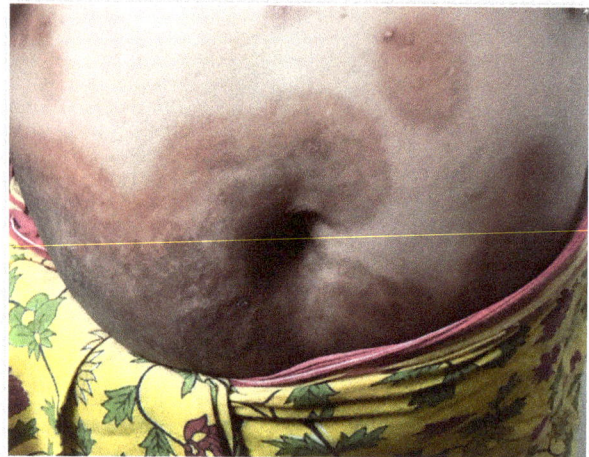

FIG. 23: Same patient as in figure 19 after complete treatment scraping negative.

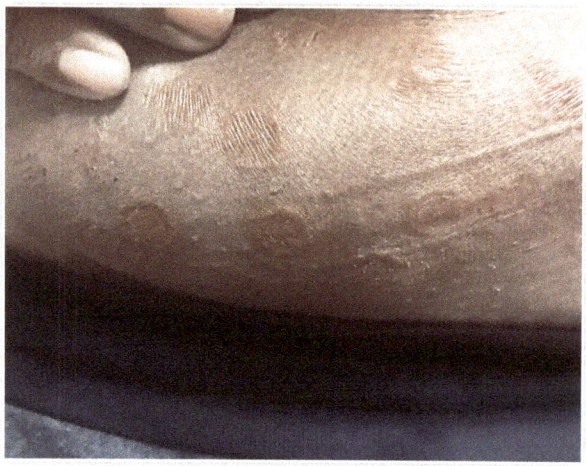

FIG. 24: Patient with insulin resistance showing involvement of multiple sites.

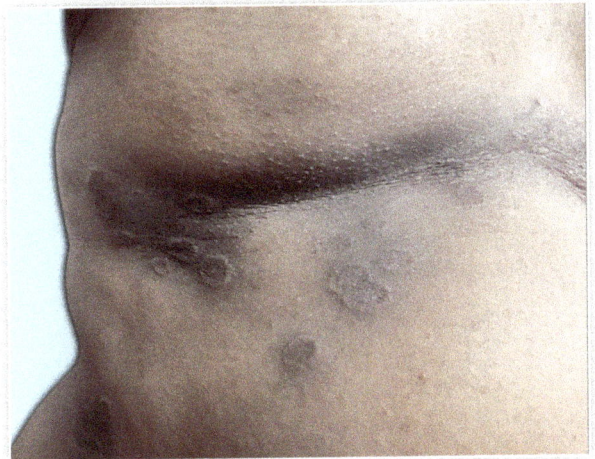

FIG. 25: Same patient as in figure 24 with more patches over the abdomen.

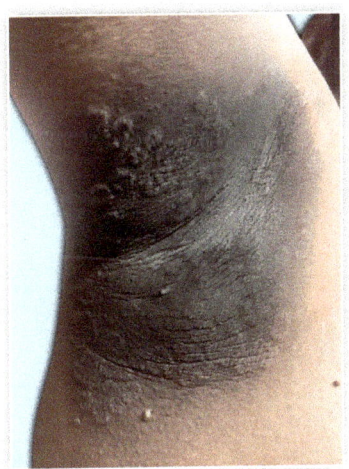

FIG. 26: Same patient as in figure 24 with patches over the axilla.

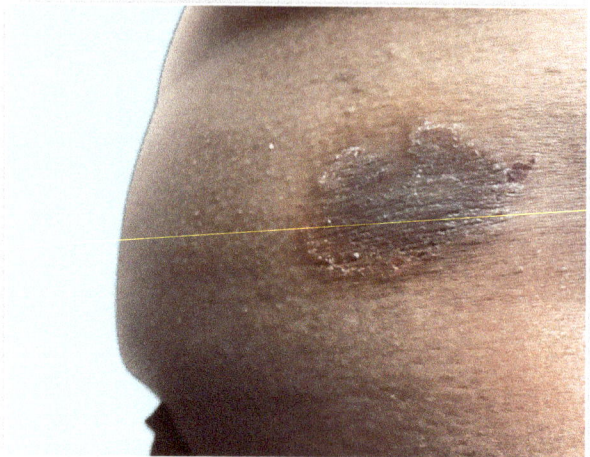

FIG. 27: Same patient as in figure 24 showing patches with raised border.

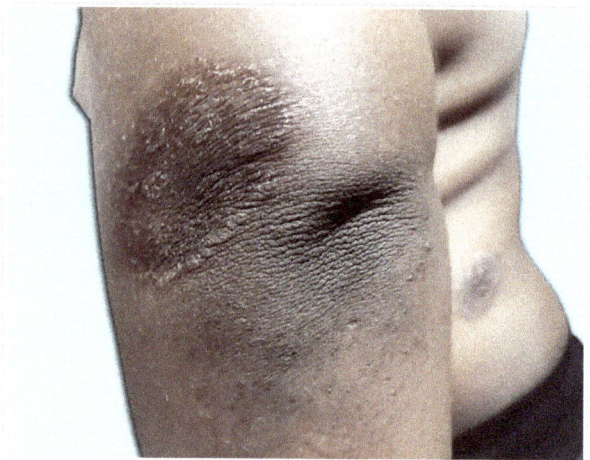

FIG. 28: Same patient as in figure 24 with extension of lesions.

Infections in the Immunocompromised

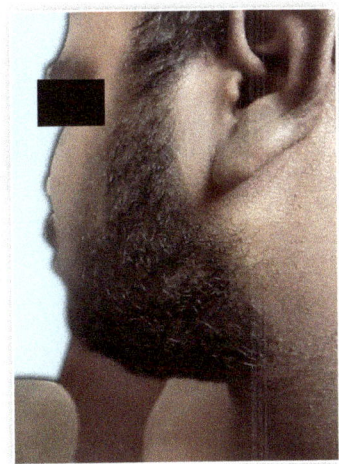

FIG. 29: Same patient as in figure 24 with facial lesions.

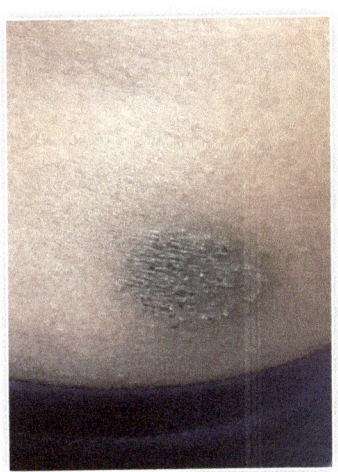

FIG. 30: Another lesion in the same patient as in figure 24.

Color Atlas of Dermatophytoses: *Focus on Superficial Fungal Infections*

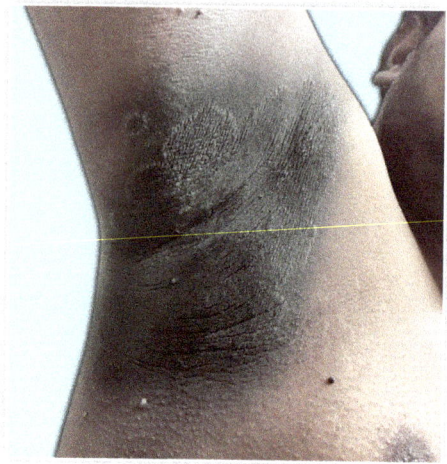

FIG. 31: Multiple site involvement in a diabetic and hypothyroid patient.

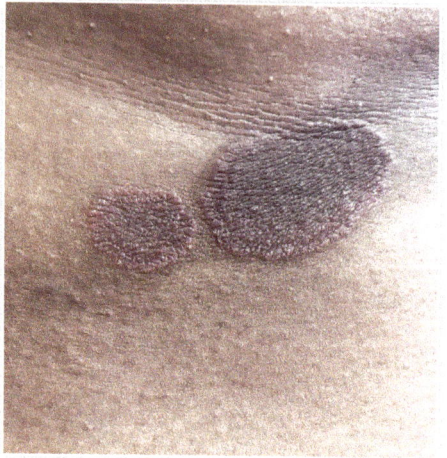

FIG. 32: Same patient as in figure 31.

Infections in the Immunocompromised

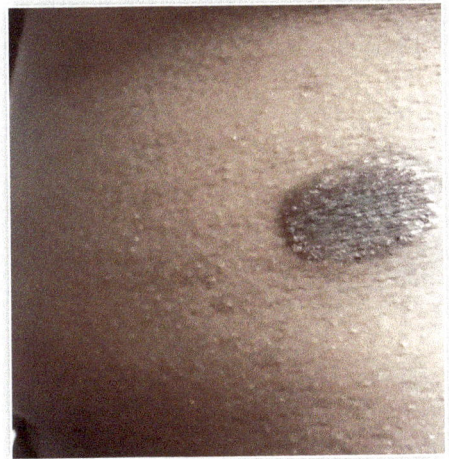

FIG. 33: Same patient as in figure 31.

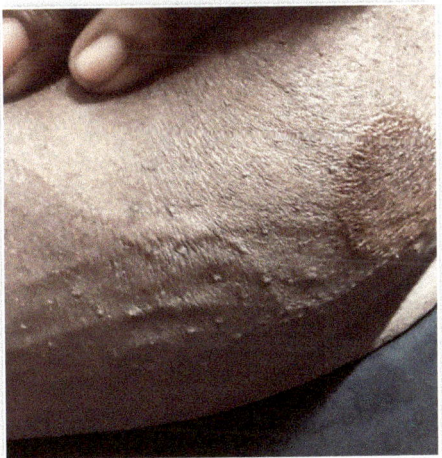

FIG. 34: Same patient as in figure 31 multiple site involvement.

Color Atlas of Dermatophytoses: *Focus on Superficial Fungal Infections*

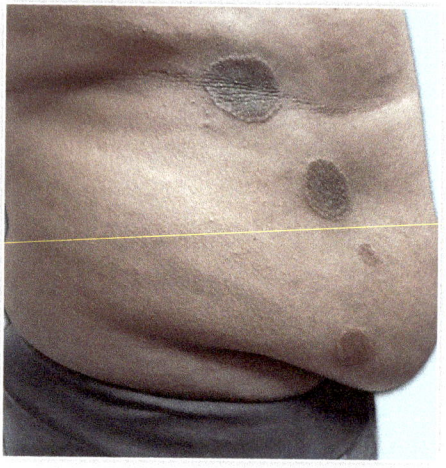

FIG. 35: Same patient as in figure 31 multiple site involvement.

CHAPTER 15: Mimickers of Dermatophytoses

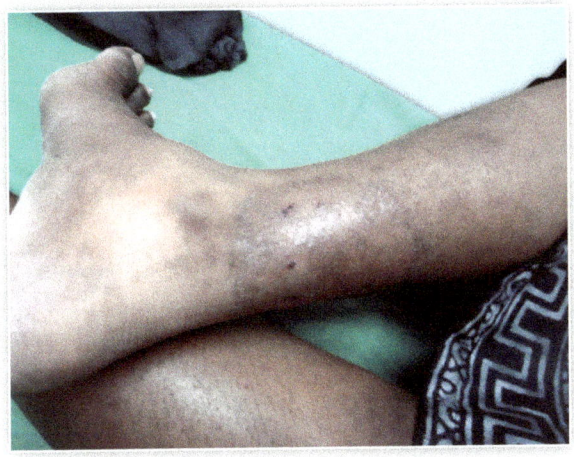

FIG. 1: Tinea corporis after topical irritant mimicking eczema.

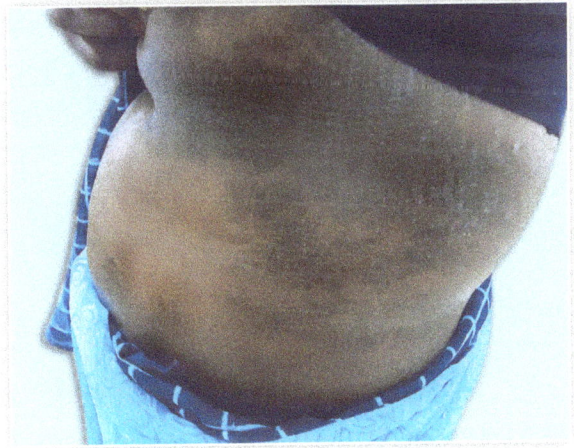

FIG. 2: Same patient as in figure 1.

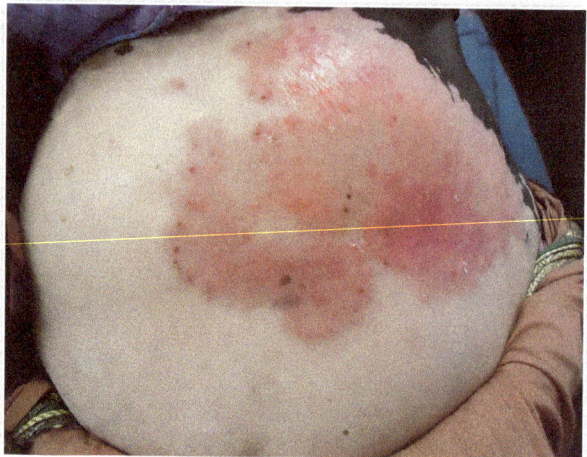

FIG. 3: Tinea corporis stopping short of the pigmented skin.

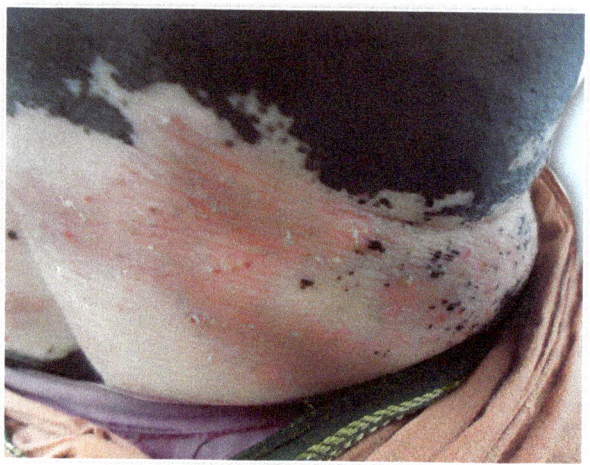

FIG. 4: Same patient as in figure 3.

Mimickers of Dermatophytoses

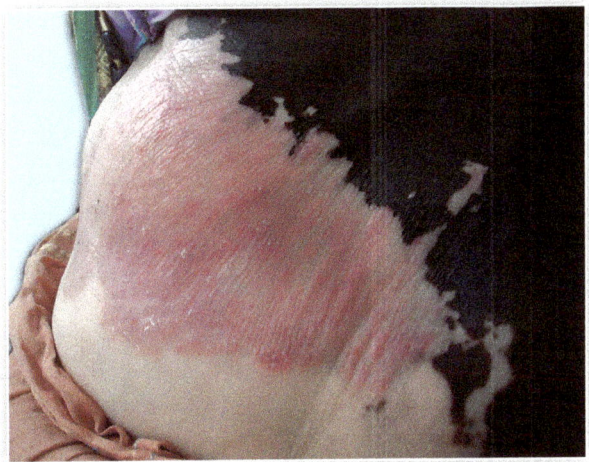

FIG. 5: Same patient as in figure 3.

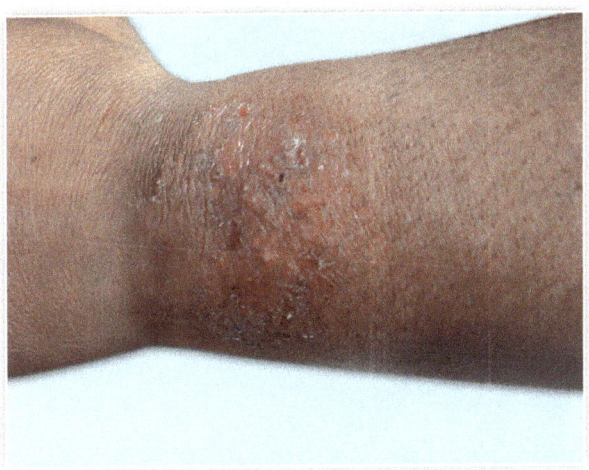

FIG. 6: Tinea corporis of the wrist resembling contact dermatitis.

Color Atlas of Dermatophytoses: *Focus on Superficial Fungal Infections*

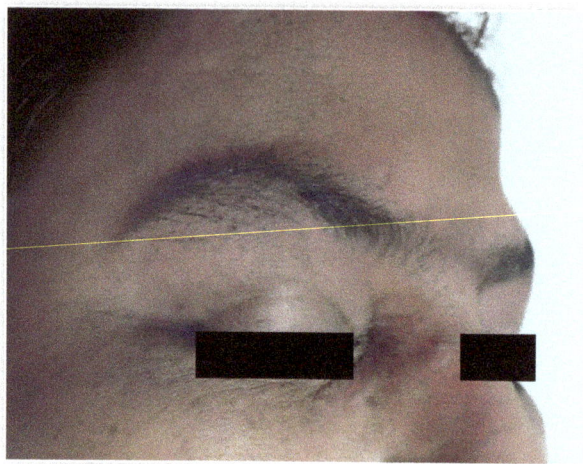

FIG. 7: Partially treated tinea corporis mimicking Hansen's disease.

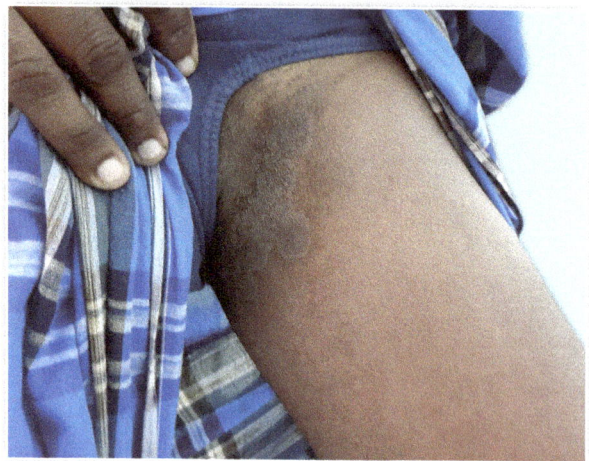

FIG. 8: Tinea cruris in a diabetic patient with intertrigo.

Mimickers of Dermatophytoses

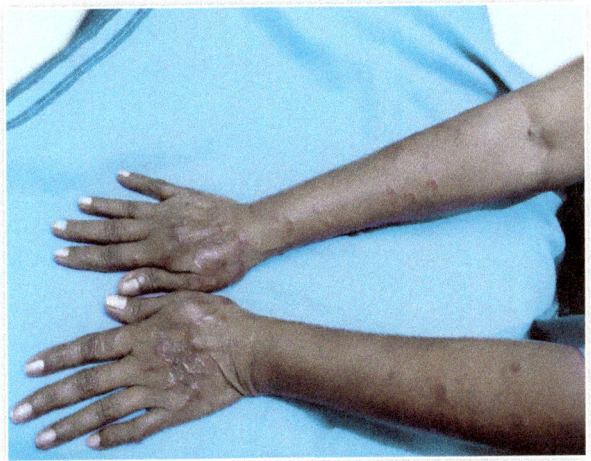

FIG. 9: Tinea corporis manuum mimicking granuloma annulare.

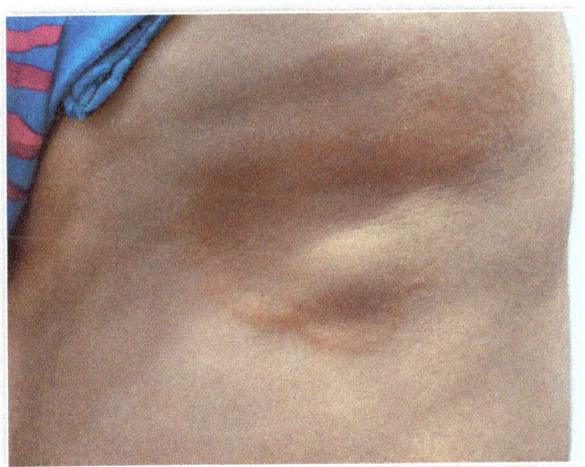

FIG. 10: Tinea corporis presenting as annular erythema.

Color Atlas of Dermatophytoses: *Focus on Superficial Fungal Infections*

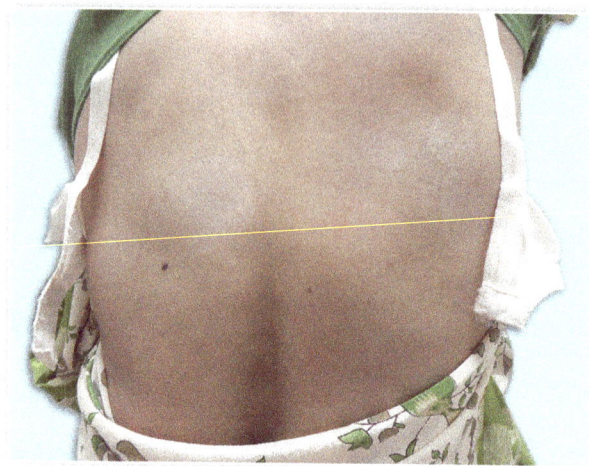

FIG. 11: Steroid combination leading to marked hypopigmentation.

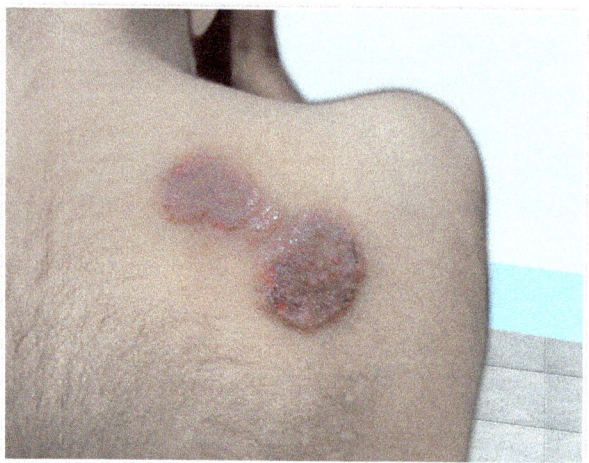

FIG. 12: Plaques of tinea corporis mimicking psoriasis.

Mimickers of Dermatophytoses

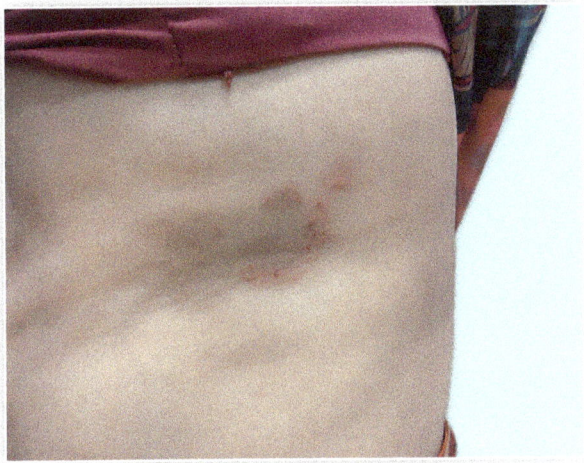

FIG. 13: Recurrence of tinea corporis mimicking cutaneous larva migrans.

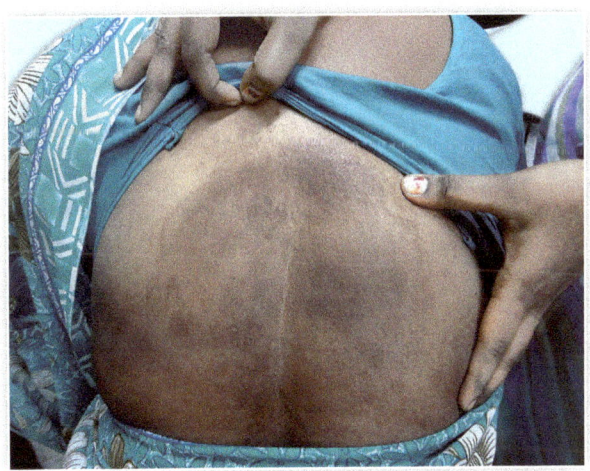

FIG. 14: Treated tinea mimicking macular amyloidosis.

Color Atlas of Dermatophytoses: *Focus on Superficial Fungal Infections*

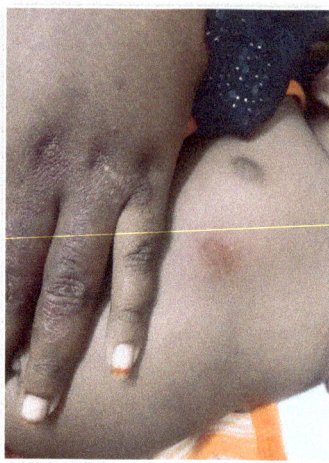

FIG. 15: Caretaker and child having dermatophyte infection.

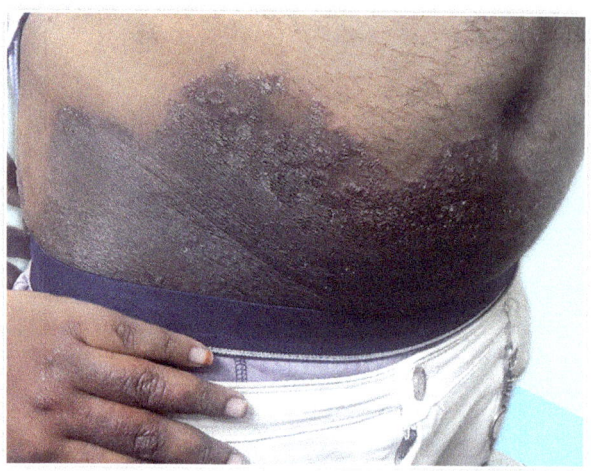

FIG. 16: With such extensive lesions, other members of the family will also get infected.

Mimickers of Dermatophytoses

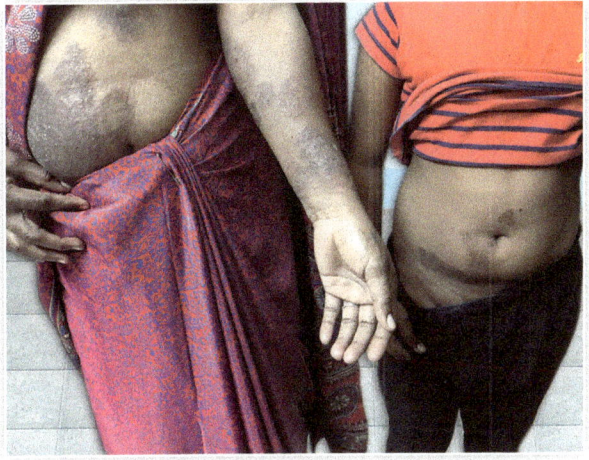

FIG. 17: Child acquiring infection from the grandmother.

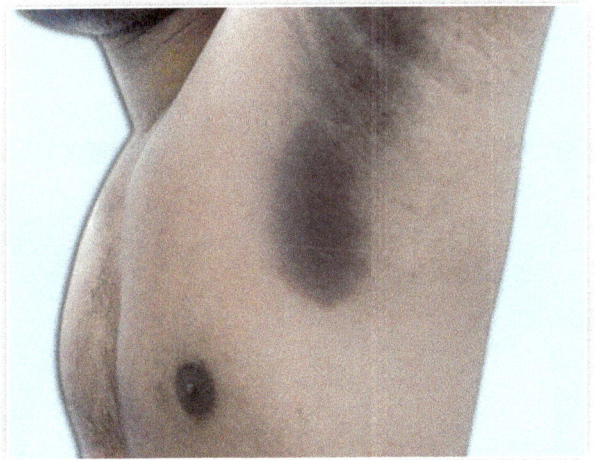

FIG. 18: Treated tinea axillaris mimicking fixed drug eruption.

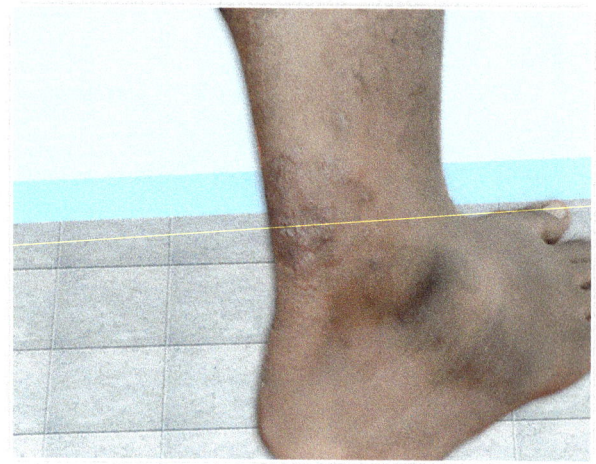

FIG. 19: Infection acquired after sharing anklet.

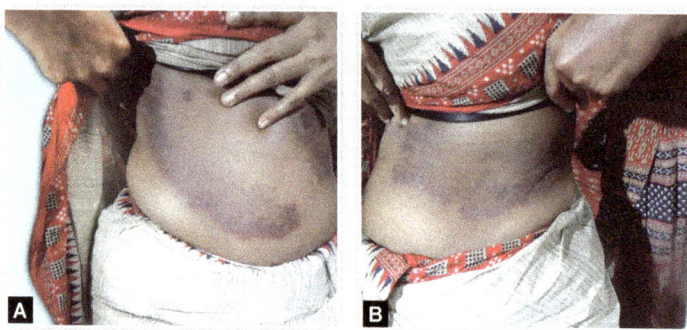

FIGS. 20A AND B: Extensive tinea corporis.

Mimickers of Dermatophytoses

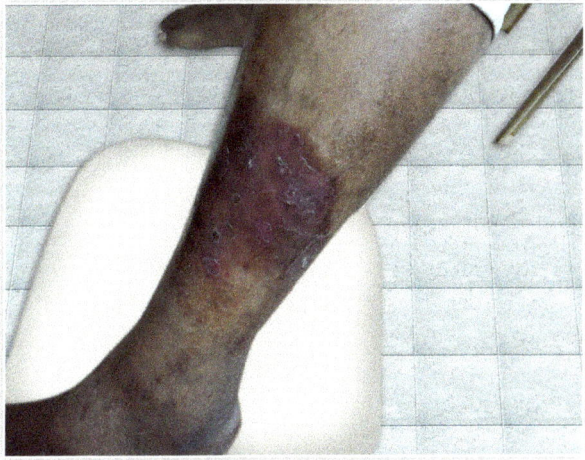

FIG. 21: Tinea over the shin in a diabetic patient mimicking NLD.

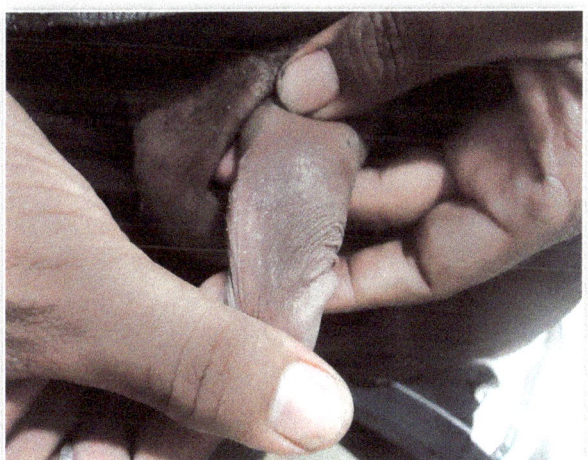

FIG. 22: Dermatophytosis mimicking lichen nitidus.

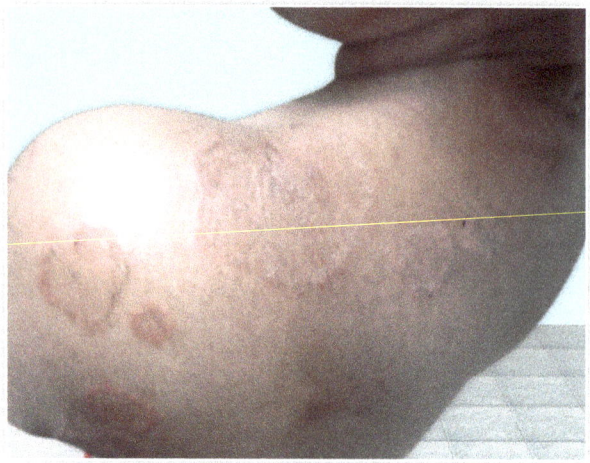

FIG. 23: Tinea corporis mimicking herald patch of pityriasis rosea.

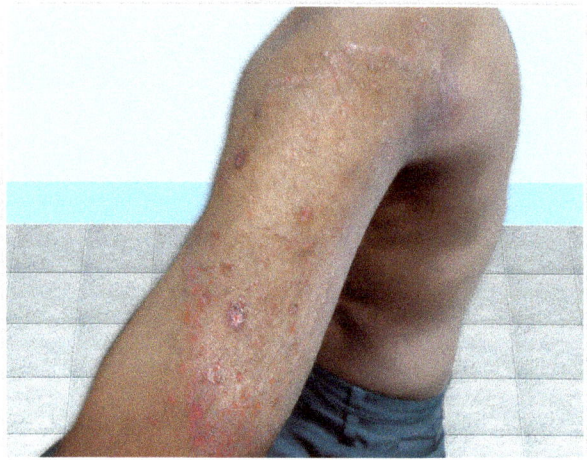

FIG. 24: Excoriations and erosions secondary to topical application in tinea corporis.

EU GSPR Authorised Reprsentative
Logos Europe, 9 rue Nicolas Poussin
1700, La Rochelle, France
Phone: +33 (0) 6 67 93 73 78
E-mail: contact@logoseurope.eu

www.ingramcontent.com/pod-product-compliance
Ingram Content Group UK Ltd.
Pitfield, Milton Keynes, MK11 3LW, UK
UKHW021827140426
5217IPUK00016B/1236